D1225395

A WOMAN DOCTOR'S GUIDE TO MENOPAUSE

A WOMAN DOCTOR'S GUIDE TO MENOPAUSE

Essential Facts and Up-to-the-Minute Information for a Woman's Change of Life

By

Dr. Lois Jovanovic, M.D. *Peterson*

with

Suzanne LeVert

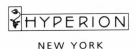

NEW YORK

This book is not intended as a substitute for medical advice of physicians and should be used only in conjunction with the advice of your personal doctor. The reader should regularly consult a physician in matters relating to his or her health and particularly with respect to any symptoms that may require diagnosis or medical attention.

LIBRARY OF CONGRESS CATALOGING-IN-PUBLICATION DATA

Jovanovic-Peterson, Lois.
    A woman doctor's guide to menopause: essential facts and up-to-the-minute information for a woman's change of life / by Lois Jovanovic with Suzanne LeVert. — 1st ed.
       p. cm.
    Includes index.
    ISBN 1-56282-855-X
    1. Menopause—Popular works. 2. Middle-aged women—Health and hygiene. I. LeVert, Suzanne. II. Title.
    RG186.J68 1993
    612.6'65—dc20   92-42739
                                        CIP

FIRST EDITION

10 9 8 7 6 5 4 3 2 1

To Charles, my husband,
and the understanding children,
Kevin, Boyce, and Larisa

—Dr. Lois Jovanovic

My thanks to Eileen Fallon
and Judith Riven for their dedicated
editorial and personal support

—Suzanne LeVert

CONTENTS

LIST OF
ILLUSTRATIONS

A WOMAN DOCTOR'S GUIDE TO MENOPAUSE

CHAPTER 1

THE MEANING OF MENOPAUSE

Menopause. Few other words in the medical lexicography have carried as much cultural, sexual, and psychological baggage as this one. For centuries, menopause was shrouded in either myth and hyperbole or utter silence. Now that women forty to sixty years of age form the fastest growing segment of the population, however, the windows of both medical science and popular culture have been opened to shed light on this once shadowy period of a woman's life. After all, despite its many peripheral implications, menopause is a quite natural physical transition that every woman will experience as she ages. In fact, by the year 2010, more than forty million American women will be at or through menopause.

If you're reading this book, chances are you're one of those forty million women. Unlike your ancestors of past centuries who died before or just after menopause, you can expect to live as much as a third of your life—a full thirty to forty years—after you are no longer fertile. This book will help you learn what to expect from this passage, how to cope with the changes that come with it, and some of the ways you can make yourself stronger and healthier before, during, and after menopause.

Like many other medical terms, the word menopause stems from Greek roots: *mens* (monthly) and *pause* (to stop). In fact, although it is commonly used to describe the whole range of symptoms that precede and follow the end of menses, the word menopause actually refers specifically to the very last menstrual period a woman experiences. Another Greek word—*klimakter*, meaning rung of the ladder—is the root of "climacteric," a term often used by gynecologists and others to describe the years before and after the menopause. Yet another word, also derived from the Greek, is "perimenopause," which means near or around menopause and, like the climacteric, is used to denote the transitional period between a woman's reproductive life and the end of her fertility. In this book, climacteric, perimenopause, and menopause will be used interchangeably, except when menopause is preceded by the word "the." In that case, "the menopause" refers specifically to the last menstrual period.

Although the age at which the menopause occurs varies from individual to individual, most women experience their last period at around the age of fifty-one. Some women menstruate throughout their fifties and into their sixties; others—about ten percent of all women—cease having their periods before the age of forty, which is considered premature menopause. Later in this chapter, we'll discuss what factors influence when a woman enters the climacteric and how you may be able to estimate when the process is likely to start in your life.

Although each woman experiences menopause in a unique way and at a different time in her life, the cause and result is the same for all of us: our ovaries eventually fail to produce the hormones we need to ripen eggs for fertilization and prepare the uterus for conception. In addition to the loss of fertility, the decrease in hormones causes or exacerbates other physical and emotional conditions common to the aging woman, including accelerated wrinkling of the skin, sagging of breast tissue, and, for some, waning of sexual desire.

Except for women who have their ovaries surgically removed (see Chapter Five), reaching the menopause is a gradual process, one that may take from five to ten years to complete. In fact, your body has been programmed to make this transition from the very moment you were conceived.

THE ANATOMY OF CHANGE

Your sex was determined at the moment of conception, when your father's sperm entered one of your mother's fallopian tubes and penetrated a mature egg, or ovum. Both the ovum and the sperm contained an equal number of carefully programmed bits of genetic material called chromosomes from each of your parents. These chromosomes determined, to a great degree, all of your physical and intellectual characteristics including, and most fundamentally, your gender.

The chromosomes that determine sex are called the XY chromosomes. The female sex is determined by the presence of two X chromosomes—one donated by each parent—while the male carries an X chromosome from his mother and a Y chromosome from his father. Because your mother was only able to contribute an X chromosome, it was the X chromosome donated by your father that determined your sex. Within eight weeks after conception, your primary sex organs—your ovaries—began to develop.

Your ovaries are a crucial part of the endocrine system, the system of the body that helps trigger and coordinate all of the body's activities, including those relating to sexuality and procreation. The endocrine system consists of several separate but interrelated glands and tissues in addition to the ovaries, including the thyroid, parathyroid, pituitary, pineal, thymus, adrenal, and pancreas. These glands and tissues secrete chemicals called hormones. Also known as the body's messengers, hormones are released into the bloodstream to deliver instructions to other organs and tissues. Virtually every bodily function—from growth and metabolism to sleep cycles and appetite—depends on hormones. The way our body uses the food we eat, for instance, depends to a large degree on the proper functioning of the hormone called insulin. Secreted into the blood by the pancreas, insulin triggers muscle, fat, and other tissues to absorb the sugar they need to fuel their activities. When the pancreas fails to produce insulin, or if the hormone does not function properly, the condition known as diabetes—high blood sugar—results.

The endocrine glands primarily responsible for sexual development, desire, and procreation are called the gonads. In men, the gonads are called testes or testicles, and these glands produce the male sex hormone testosterone. In women, the gonads are the ovaries, two glands comprised of smooth muscle located in the lower abdomen, one on each side of the uterus, also known as the womb (see Figure 1, page 20). The ovaries produce and store eggs, as well as secrete the female sex hormones, estrogen and progesterone. In addition to the primary gonads, estrogen is also produced by the adrenal glands, which are located on top of each kidney.

Although it may come as a surprise to you, the female body also produces and uses a certain amount of male sex hormones. Both the adrenal glands and the ovaries produce small amounts of androgens (testosterone and androstenedione) and deliver them into the bloodstream. These androgens influence the growth of pubic and other body hair in women and also appear to influence a woman's sex drive. In addition, the body is able to transform some androgens into estrogen through a conversion process that takes place in certain fat cells.

From birth to adolescence, ovarian activity is fairly dormant. Although a child grows and changes in many other ways, physical sexual development does not usually begin until she reaches the average age of eight to ten years. At that time, an internal alarm clock in the brain, most likely triggered by the young girl's body weight and percentage of body fat, signals the start of puberty by stimulating the ovaries to produce the sex hormones, estrogen and progesterone, as well as small amounts of androgens. Among the most powerful chemicals known to man or woman, these sex hormones provoke several physical changes to take place. Known as secondary sex characteristics, these developments include the budding of breasts, the growth of pubic and underarm hair, increasing height and weight, and dermatological changes. About two years after these changes first begin to occur, the young girl reaches menarche and menstruates for the first time.

For most young girls, the menstrual period is the most dramatic representation of her emerging womanhood. Indeed, the menstrual cycle quickly becomes an integral part of every young woman's life and remains one until the onset of menopause some thirty to forty years later. Nevertheless, few of us fully understand the process of menstruation or appreciate what a truly remarkable work of nature our reproductive system is.

THE MENSTRUAL CYCLE

A female child is born with ovaries that are completely stocked with all the eggs she will ever have—about one million. During her fertile life, a woman will release just three hundred to four hundred eggs—one each month for about thirty-five to forty years. The rest simply atrophy. As menopause commences, only about ten thousand eggs remain.

Each egg, which is little more than a dot of fluid packed with genetic information, is encapsulated in a tiny sac called a follicle and lodged within ovarian tissue. Every month, your body prepares one egg (and occasionally two) for fertilization and the uterus for a potential pregnancy. This preparation is what is known as the menstrual cycle. Although by definition a cycle has no beginning or end, for descriptive purposes we will assign the starting position of the menstrual cycle to the hypothalamus, an endocrine gland in the brain. At the beginning of the cycle, the hypothamalus sends a message in the form of a hormone called gonadotropin-releasing hormone (GnRH) to the pituitary gland. The pituitary, which is located just below the hypothalamus, then relays its own message to the ovaries by another hormone called the follicle-stimulating hormone (FSH).

Stimulation from FSH causes one of the follicles in one of the ovaries to grow and the ovum within it to mature. At the same time, a thick layer of cells covers the follicle and ovum; these cells secrete the hormone estradiol, a type of estrogen. The estrogen is released into the bloodstream and acts on the lining of the uterus, called the endometrium, causing it to grow and thicken in preparation for the arrival of a fertilized egg. This occurs during the first part of the cycle, called the estrogen phase, which takes about fourteen days.

At this time, the hypothalamus, stimulated by the elevated levels of estrogen in the bloodstream, signals the pituitary to secrete a second hormone, known as luteinizing hormone (LH). The surge of LH causes the developing follicle to enlarge and rupture. In an event known as ovulation, the mature ovum is then expelled into the fallopian tubes and makes its way up into the uterus, a journey that takes about six days. While it is in transit, the egg can be fertilized if sperm are present.

In the meantime, the remnant follicle in the ovary is transformed into a working endocrine gland called the corpus luteum. The corpus luteum produces both estrogen and large quantities of progesterone, the female hormone that is dominant in the second half of the cycle, known as the luteal phase. Under the impact of progesterone, the cells in the uterine lining grow and mature further. By the end of the menstrual cycle, the endometrium has doubled in thickness, and large amounts of nutrients meant to nourish a fetus have been stored there.

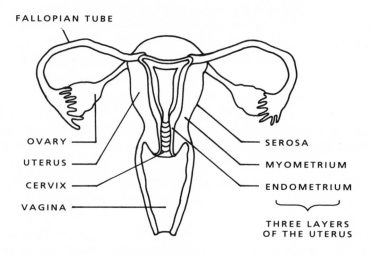

FIGURE 1   Female reproductive organs.

If the egg is fertilized by a sperm, the fertilized egg implants itself into the lining of the endometrium and a special hormone, called chorionic gonadotrophin, is secreted to stimulate the continued production of estrogen and progesterone. In fact, the egg itself becomes its very own hormone-producing factory. Without fertilization and continued hormone secretion, the corpus luteum begins to shrink and levels of estrogen and progesterone drop. When the hormonal level is at its lowest, the uterus sheds its lining and what is known as the menstrual period begins. By the fourth or fifth day of the period, hormonal levels have dropped enough to signal the hypothalamus to resume the process. Unless interrupted by pregnancy, surgical removal of the ovaries, or a hormonal imbalance caused by illness or stress, this remarkable cycle continues throughout a woman's fertile life.

THE CLIMACTERIC

The average woman of the late twentieth century is fertile for about thirty to forty years. As early as her midthirties, however, her hormonal cycle may begin to change and her fertility to diminish. Not only has her store of eggs been severely depleted, but the follicles that remain are less sensitive to hormonal stimulation from the FSH and LH sent by the hypothalamus and the pituitary gland. Some months, one follicle is aroused enough to ripen and release an egg; other months, no ovulation occurs. This stage of a woman's reproductive life, when the ovaries gradually decrease their function and periods become irregular, is called premenopause. During premenopause, you may menstruate more often or less often, skip periods altogether, or have heavier or lighter than usual periods.

Without the release of an egg during ovulation, progesterone, which depends on the empty follicle (corpus luteum) for production, is no longer secreted at all. Although estrogen levels also drop, the ovaries, adrenal glands, and fat cells are still able to produce some estrogen. The uterine lining, then, is being stimulated exclusively by estrogen. It continues to grow until it lacks a sufficient blood supply, which can take several months; not only does the woman miss one or two periods, but when she does shed the endometrium, it often results in a much heavier period than usual. At this time, she may begin to experience some of the symptoms and side-effects of this decrease in estrogen and progesterone, such as hot flashes, as well. These symptoms will be covered in depth in Chapter Two.

Meanwhile, the original triggers of the cycle, the hypothalamus and pituitary gland, continue to release FSH and LH in an increasingly futile attempt to stimulate ovarian activity. In fact, the level of FSH can reach thirteen times its norm, and LH levels triple during this time—a sure sign to a gynecologist that the patient has entered the climacteric. Eventually, the ovarian follicles no longer respond to hormonal prodding and menopause is achieved. After a woman has gone for a full year without menstruating, menopause is complete and she enters the postmenopausal phase of her life.

HOT FLASH!

Early menopause does not have to mean the end of fertility for all women. Although a woman no longer produces eggs after menopause, her uterus—the womb—is still viable. Hormonal therapy taken before and during pregnancy allows a woman to carry a fetus, created through in-vitro fertilization using her spouse's sperm and a donated egg, to full term. In fact, this process may present no age barrier: the most recent case involves a fifty-two-year-old woman.

It may surprise you to learn that the ovaries still produce some estrogen after menopause, as do the adrenal glands. Perhaps even more surprising is that the androgens—the male sex hormones—that have been produced all along by both the ovaries and the adrenals, play a much larger role than ever before in maintaining a woman's hormonal health. Once estrogen reaches a low level, certain fat cells are stimulated to take up the androgens circulating in the blood and convert them to estrone, a weak form of estrogen. Although the amount of this type of estrogen will not be sufficient for fertility, it may alleviate some symptoms of menopause.

INFLUENCES ON MENOPAUSE

For most modern American women, the last menstrual period usually occurs between the ages of 45 and 55, with the median age being 51.4 years. Since the beginning of the century, both the age of the menopause and the average life expectancy has increased by about four years. Improved nutrition, better living conditions, and better overall health among women are seen as the most likely explanations for the increased years of fertility now experienced by today's Americans.

HOT FLASH!

A woman living in 1693 had a less than 30 percent chance of surviving past menopause. Today, three hundred years later, women will live more than a third of their lives after they are no longer fertile.

The age at which an individual reaches menopause is a highly individual matter. Indeed, every woman seems to have her own internal hormonal clock that signals the beginning and end of her reproductive life. Contrary to popular belief, the age at which you first started to menstruate *does not* affect the age at which you pass through menopause, nor does the number of children you have had, or whether or not you have taken oral contraceptives. Although predicting exactly when you, as an individual, will enter the climacteric is impossible, there are several factors that influence at what age you'll be at the menopause and how your body will react to the change.

Heredity

There is some evidence that a predisposition to early or late menopause may be inherited. Whether such a tendency is due to genetic factors or to shared environmental conditions such as diet, stress, and other lifestyle factors is still controversial. Asking your mother about her menopause experience may give you some insight about what your own experience may be like.

Diet

It appears that the better nourished women are, the later they experience menopause. Studies conducted in New Guinea during the 1970s and published in England, for instance, found that undernourished women entered the climacteric at about age forty-three, while those more adequately nourished passed through the menopause about four years later. Both better nutrition, (i.e., a more balanced diet) and heavier body weight (see below) contribute to these statistics.

Weight

If you are extremely thin, you have a greater chance of experiencing an early menopause and suffering more symptoms of menopause than someone who is overweight. This is primarily due to the fact that fatty tissue is able to secrete estrogen, increasing the body's supply of this essential hormone. (This fact does *not* warrant a weight gain solely to avoid menopause; the problems associated with obesity are more serious than those that may accompany menopause.)

Smoking

All other factors being equal, a woman who smokes more than half a pack of cigarettes a day will undergo menopause from five to ten years earlier than other members of her family. Although the reason for this is not yet fully understood, it is believed that nicotine, which acts on the central nervous system, may both decrease the secretion and lower the performance of hormones. Smoking also increases the risk of osteoporosis—one of the most common and serious side-effects of menopause and aging—by reducing the thickness of bone. (See Chapter Three.)

Surgery

The most widespread cause of early menopause is the surgical removal of both ovaries, called a bilateral oophorectomy. This loss of your ovaries—usually along with your uterus and cervix—causes a sudden and dramatic loss of most of your sex hormones. Menopause occurs immediately, no matter what your age.

Autoimmune disorder

In extremely rare cases, a woman's own immune system may turn against the cells of the ovaries and destroy healthy cells, thereby provoking an early menopause.

Abnormal chromosomes

Also quite rare is the woman born with a chromosomal disorder causing her to have dramatically fewer eggs than normal. This woman would simply run out of ova before she reaches the average age for menopause.

Chemotherapy/radiation

The good news is that more and more women are surviving cancer today than ever before. Unfortunately, the chemotherapy and/or radiation treatments required to kill the proliferating cells often disrupt or destroy healthy tissue as well, including ovarian tissue responsible for producing estrogen and progesterone. Women who undergo such treatment for cancer may find themselves experiencing menopause much earlier than they may have otherwise. Adding insult to injury, the resulting symptoms tend to be more severe and unpredictable than those suffered by women who experience a natural menopause.

Keeping in mind these general exceptions, you can expect to start the process of menopause anytime after the age of forty. Along with irregular or changed periods, you may experience several other symptoms as ovarian function continues to decline. These symptoms include not only the infamous hot flashes, but, for some women, fatigue, irritability, decrease in sexual desire, and skin changes that include dryness of the vagina, tingling sensations, and increased wrinkling of facial skin. In addition to these annoying but usually benign symptoms, loss of estrogen may also have long-term, serious side effects, including increased risk of heart disease and osteoporosis.

Before we launch into a full discussion of these symptoms and side-effects in Chapter Two, let's dispel some of the myths that still surround menopause today.

THE MYTHS OF MENOPAUSE

"Menopause will make me old."

"Menopause will make me fat."

"Menopause will make me crazy or depressed."

"Menopause means having to take drugs."
"Menopause means a hysterectomy."
"Having problems during menopause means I'm inadequate."

No doubt you've heard these rumors, and even if you don't completely believe them, there is probably a part of you that fears that one or more of them may be true for you. Take heart: these common myths about menopause are largely unfounded. On the other hand, like many rumors, there may be a grain of truth to at least some of them. Let's take them one by one:

MYTH 1 Menopause will make me old

At the same time you lose your fertility, other signs of aging will, no doubt, occur. Your hair may start to turn grey; your body weight may shift as gravity finally gains some ground in its forty or fifty year battle with your breasts, abdomen, and derriere; your skin may begin to wrinkle more quickly and deeply than ever before. Your sleep patterns may be altered and you'll require fewer or more hours of rest to feel refreshed. However, you *cannot* hold menopause solely and absolutely responsible for all of these changes.

In fact, although lack of estrogen may be responsible for some dermatological changes and for more serious problems such as osteoporosis and heart disease, other symptoms of advancing age are unrelated to female hormonal activity. More to the point, if you think these changes inevitably come with menopause, you're likely to simply accept them. But there are several steps you can take—medically, nutritionally, physically, and cosmetically—that will keep you feeling younger and healthier for longer than ever before...if you follow them.

MYTH 2 Menopause will make me fat

Estrogen and progesterone have little, if any, effect on the way your body metabolizes food. Therefore, the loss of these hormones during and after menopause should not result in any significant weight gain. However, there is some evidence that because the balance between female hormones and androgens—male hormones—has been disturbed, body weight may be redistributed: breasts and buttocks may lose fatty tissue while the abdomen gains fat, causing some women to acquire the midsection fat more common in men. In addition, poor muscle tone of the stomach also can cause sagging.

Although an excess of male hormones may be partly responsible for the dreaded "middle-age spread," the real culprit is our lifestyle. As a woman ages, she tends to exercise less while eating the same amount of food—or more. In addition, older women generally need *fewer* calories to fulfill their body's need for nutrition than they did when they were younger. In fact, the average basal metabolic rate of a menopausal woman is about 20 percent lower than women who still menstruate. However, you can prevent gaining weight after menopause by following a healthy eating plan and exercising regularly. (See Chapters Seven and Eight.)

| MYTH 3 | Menopause will make me crazy or depressed

The drop in estrogen and progesterone may cause mood swings and irritability for a short time. As you'll read in Chapter Four, treatment with estrogen and progesterone may help alleviate these symptoms. However, whether or not the full spectrum of psychological or emotional symptoms accompanying menopause are directly due to the lack of female hormones remains controversial. For most women, the transition from fertility to postmenopause comes at a time when other major changes are occurring simultaneously. Children may be leaving home, careers changing or ending, marriages breaking up or under strain as both partners come face to face with aging. These stresses may be just as responsible for emotional upheavals as the hormonal imbalance posed by menopause.

Indeed, a recent study, published in the January 1992 issue of the British journal *Maturitas*, followed 477 pre- and postmenopausal women in Winnipeg, Manitoba for five years. The authors of the study, Doctors P.A. Kaufert, P. Gilbert, and R. Tate, found that issues such as their children leaving home, the illness and/or death of other family members, and their own health problems put these women at far greater risk for depression than any hormonal changes accompanying menopause.

The good news is that despite the enormous stresses upon women as they enter the climacteric, we are all probably stronger than we think. Very few women experience clinical depression requiring medication during menopause, and among those who do, underlying psychological problems are usually present before the loss of female hormones. Keep in mind that the mood swings and depression you may feel are very real and may indeed have a hormonal basis. But the very fact that any depression experienced during menopause may not be physically determined should encourage you to fight against it with everything you've got. Exercising regularly, eating a healthy diet, and taking the time to pamper yourself are three ways to push the "middle-age" blues away.

MYTH 4 | Menopause means taking drugs

Although recent medical advances have made hormone replacement therapy (HRT) safe and available to more women than ever before, these drugs are not for everyone. Women with some types of breast cancer, fibroid tumors, and blood disorders should discuss HRT carefully with their doctors. HRT also has risks and side effects that must be weighed against the severity of your symptoms before you decide to partake of them. Many women pass through menopause with only minimal symptoms and do not feel the need for medical intervention. However, if you are uncomfortable—physically or emotionally—chances are good that you'll benefit from some form of hormonal replacement. (See Chapter Four for more information.)

MYTH 5 | Menopause means hysterectomy

Actually, this myth is two misconceptions rolled into one. First, many women assume that having a hysterectomy means automatic menopause. In fact, as we'll discuss in Chapter Four, there are several different kinds of hysterectomies and only one of them—a bilateral oophorectomy or total hysterectomy—means certain menopause. A simple hysterectomy on the other hand, involves removal of only the uterus and cervix. Although the after-effects of this surgery are often quite uncomfortable and unsettling, most women are still able to produce estrogen on a regular cycle.

Second, until recently, many doctors rather callously believed that once women had passed through menopause, they had no need for their "reproductive equipment" and encouraged women to have total hysterectomies. To be fair, physicians felt that the risks of developing ovarian and uterine cancer were great enough to justify surgery in a postmenopausal woman who displayed any abnormal symptoms, such as uterine bleeding or fibroids. Thanks in large part to the current focus on women's health and health advocacy, the risks and benefits of this controversial surgery are being weighed far more carefully. Menopause no longer means hysterectomy, and vice versa, in more and more cases every day.

BEST BET!

Learn about the special risks you, as a woman approaching or past menopause, have for osteoporosis, heart disease, diabetes, arthritis, and other conditions common in older adults and how to prevent them from developing. It's the best first step you can take to assure that the final third of your life is the healthiest and most active one yet.

MENOPAUSE AND YOUR HEALTH

To reiterate a point made at the beginning of this chapter, it is likely that you will live more than a third of your life after menopause. No longer does "the change of life" mean the "end of life." In fact, many women find that once the stresses of childbearing (to say nothing of childrearing!) have been relieved after menopause, they find themselves feeling better and more energetic than they did when they were younger. New jobs, new interests, better sex—even better health—follow the menopause for more women than ever before. Indeed, we can now see menopause for what it truly is: simply another milestone along a woman's path through life.

Keeping that in mind may help you as you approach or pass through menopause. To do so in good health and with vigor will no doubt take some effort and commitment on your part. The physical decline that eventually comes with aging is an inevitable and natural part of life, but there are ways to make your later years ones filled with physical, intellectual, and emotional energy and well-being.

CHAPTER 2

MENOPAUSE: SIGNS AND SYMPTOMS

Your Premenopause Self-Test

Answer the following questions with a yes or no to see if you may be experiencing symptoms related to approaching menopause.

1) Are you missing periods? _____
2) Is your cycle irregular? _____
3) Are your periods closer together or further apart than in the past?____
4) Are you bleeding more heavily or lightly than in the past? ____
5) Are you spotting between periods? ____
6) If you have experienced premenstrual syndrome in the past, have those symptoms changed or worsened? Are you experiencing any of the following symptoms for the first time?

      _____ breast tenderness

      _____ nausea

      _____ cramping

      _____ abdominal pain

      _____ weight gain

      _____ headaches

      _____ irritability

      _____ lethargy or exhaustion

      _____ sadness or depression

7) Do you have an itch or irritation in the vaginal area?____
8) Is your vagina dry during intercourse?____
9) Do you experience sudden waves of heat, perspiration, or redness of the skin?____
10) Are you approaching the age when your mother passed through menopause?____

If you're nearing the average age for menopause (about fifty-one), the more questions you answered with a "yes," the more likely it is that your ovaries are beginning to decline in function and you are no longer producing adequate estrogen or progesterone. In any case, if you are experiencing significant changes in your menstrual cycle, particularly missed periods, heavy bleeding, or abdominal pain, it is essential that you see your gynecologist as soon as possible. Although menopause may indeed be the culprit, other conditions, including cancer, fibroids, and hormonal disorders must be ruled out.

As soon as other possible causes are eliminated, diagnosing menopause is usually quite simple. Your gynecologist will ask you questions about your menstrual cycle similar to the ones listed above, review your past medical history, and perhaps perform one or both of the following tests. The FSH (follicle stimulating hormone) test is a simple blood test that measures the level of FSH, which, as you may remember from Chapter One, rises sharply at the beginning of the cycle in order to stimulate the ovary to produce estrogen. If estrogen is not produced, the hypothalamus and pituitary gland continue to secrete FSH to up to thirteen times the norm following your final period. If you are over forty and experiencing menopausal symptoms, particularly irregular periods, and your FSH level is even slightly elevated, your gynecologist may assume that you have entered the climacteric.

Another test measures how much estrogen you are secreting into your vaginal tissue. This test entails scraping the upper walls of the vagina; in fact, it is often done at the same time as a routine Pap smear. Although less accurate than the FSH test in predicting or diagnosing menopause, the vaginal smear may be helpful in assessing the cause of sexual dysfunction, particularly painful intercourse, which can be exacerbated by lack of estrogen. And, as you'll learn in Chapter Four, some gynecologists now recommend the test to women during their early forties, even *before* they exhibit signs of hormonal decline. That way, if they later decide to take hormone replacement therapy, their doctors can prescribe a dose of estrogen that will more accurately match their own natural, premenopause estrogen level.

More than likely, however, the tests your doctor performs will merely confirm an obvious diagnosis, especially if you are in your late forties or early fifties. No doubt you will experience one or more telltale physical and emotional symptoms caused by your fluctuating and diminishing hormonal levels. How subtle or severe these symptoms are varies greatly from individual to individual (see Table 1, below). Some women pass through the climacteric smoothly and easily; others are plagued with uncomfortable and upsetting symptoms.

TABLE 1

Signs and Symptoms of Menopause

Menstrual changes

Hot flashes

Sleep disturbances

Dermatological changes (skin and hair)

Formication (tingling sensations)

Vaginal atrophy (dryness and infections)

Urinary tract disturbances

Mood swings or depression

Sex drive changes

Long-Term Complications

Osteoporosis

Cardiovascular Disease

The difference between those who have an easy time and those who have more difficulty is largely the rate at which they stop producing estrogen: women whose estrogen levels drop suddenly and dramatically (including those who undergo the surgical removal of their ovaries) are likely to suffer far more serious symptoms than those women who lose ovarian function gradually, over several months or years. Heavy women also may have an easier time with symptoms than thin women because they have more fatty tissue with which to manufacture additional estrogen.

Whether you suffer mild symptoms or more dramatic ones, you'll no doubt be unnerved, at least a bit, during this phase of your life. As you enter the climacteric, it may be helpful for you to reflect upon your own experience during puberty, since both of these natural transitions involve hormonal changes with striking physical and emotional symptoms. No doubt you remember how awkward and confused you felt during those years when your body seemed to both transform and betray you. As a young adolescent, your periods were probably irregular, your moods equally unpredictable, and your skin subject to disruptions of oil, acne, or dryness. As an adult approaching menopause, you may display the same or quite similar symptoms—and you may feel just as awkward and embarrassed! Keep in mind that both the changes you experience and the feelings you have about them are perfectly natural.

MENSTRUAL CHANGES

The hallmark sign of perimenopause—the time span of about five to ten years before the last period—is a change in the menstrual cycle. As described in Chapter One, this change occurs because the ovaries gradually lose their ability to ripen and release eggs and to produce the female sex hormones, estrogen and progesterone. As that happens, your periods become irregular.

Some women notice that both the interval between their periods and the amount of menstrual flow *decreases* as ovarian function declines. During a normal period, menstrual flow begins when the level of estrogen drops because an egg has not been fertilized in the uterus. At this point, the uterine lining dies and menstrual flow occurs. During perimenopause, however, the endometrium often fails to fully mature due to lack of sufficient hormonal stimulation. In this case, menstruation may take place earlier—every twenty-one instead of every twenty-eight days, for instance—and the flow may be lighter than usual.

Other women find that they menstruate less often but their flow is extremely heavy. One reason such a pattern could evolve is that a woman is failing to ovulate at all. Without the release of an egg, the corpus luteum cannot exist to produce progesterone, since it arises from an empty follicle. Although estrogen continues to be secreted at a normal level, progesterone production has ceased altogether, leaving the uterine lining to grow under continuous estrogen stimulation for long periods of time. When estrogen production finally stops for that cycle, the period is usually much heavier and lasts longer than it did before perimenopause.

Many women entering the climacteric also experience spotting between periods or just before the start of their periods. This is a signal that the uterus is receiving mixed messages from all four of the hormones—FSH, LH, estrogen, and progesterone—associated with the menstrual cycle. Once working together in meticulous harmony, they are now erratically produced and in an unbalanced state.

Some women exhibit no specific pattern in their menstrual changes. One month the period is heavy, the next it is light, and periods arrive and subside almost randomly. Eventually, ovulation will cease completely and you will no longer have periods at all; this usually happens at about the age of about fifty-one or fifty-two. Very few women still menstruate after the age of fifty-four.

As soon as you notice that your periods have become irregular, keep careful track of your symptoms. Write down when your periods start, how long they last, and if you notice any changes in flow, then bring the log to your next appointment with your gynecologist. It will help him or her decide what, if any, treatment you may require to help smooth out your periods. *Remember, if you are bleeding between periods and have not yet seen your doctor, make an appointment right away to rule out other causes.*

If the irregularity of your periods is particularly troublesome or if you tend to build up so much endometrial tissue that your periods are extremely heavy, your gynecologist may prescribe progesterone therapy, which replaces the progesterone you would produce if you were ovulating. For one or two weeks a month, you'll take a progesterone tablet, which will help to counteract the buildup of the endometrium. When you stop taking the pills, the resulting lack of progesterone will induce a period. Taken in this manner, progesterone tablets help to regulate your cycles and make sure that your endometrium is shed every month. Eventually, when you run out of sufficient estrogen to cause the lining to build up every month, your periods will stop even if you continue to take progesterone. (More about progesterone in Chapter Four.)

WHAT ELSE COULD IT BE?

Although the onset of menopause is the most likely explanation for irregular periods in women over the age of forty-five, there may be other reasons for these symptoms. In fact—believe it or not—you could be pregnant, even if your periods have been erratic for several months. Ovulation still occurs, albeit less often, in the perimenopausal stage, and it is possible that you could produce an egg that becomes fertilized. For that reason, using some form of birth control is essential for at least a year following your last period if you wish to avoid an unwanted pregnancy.

There are also several benign—and not so benign—reasons for missed periods, spotting, or heavy bleeding. They include endometrial hyperplasia (an overgrowth of endometrial tissue that could be early sign of cancer), fibroids (noncancerous tumors), polyps (small, benign tumors on the uterus), endometriosis (the growth of endometrial tissue outside the uterus), or a cancer of the reproductive organs. Most of these conditions are easily treated, but others may require surgery or other medical intervention. If you have been diagnosed with any of these conditions, please read Chapter Five carefully to ascertain your options for treatment.

HOT FLASHES

The most common side effect of menopause, suffered by at least 75 percent of menopausal women, is the hot flash. Although every woman who's had a hot flash describes it in a slightly different way, it generally involves a sudden rush of heat to the upper body that starts in the chest area and spreads to the arms, neck, and face. The skin reddens and may feel hot to the touch. In many instances, the flush is accompanied by a rapid heartbeat (up to 10 to 15 percent faster than normal), shallow breathing, and heavy perspiration. Hot flashes can occur infrequently or, in severe cases, up to fifty times a day. They last anywhere from three to five minutes each, with rare cases lasting thirty minutes or more. The after-effects of hot flash episodes include exhaustion, chills, and a tightness of the skin that may continue for several hours.

As unpleasant as hot flashes may be to the women who experience them, they are, in fact, a harmless reaction to the hormonal imbalance. As you may remember from Chapter One, the trigger for the start of the reproductive cycle is the release of a hormone (GnRH) from the hypothalamus, a region of the brain. The hypothalamus releases this hormone when the level of estrogen produced by the ovaries falls to a certain low level, signalling to certain cells—called estrogen receptors—that an egg has not been fertilized and another reproductive cycle should begin. Triggered by GnRH, the pituitary then secretes its own pair of powerful hormones, FSH and LH.

In addition to menstruation, however, the hypothalamus and the pituitary act as command centers for several other basic body functions, including temperature, thirst, hunger, water balance, and sexual functioning. The hypothalamus, for instance, is one of the endocrine glands responsible for secreting norepinephrine, a hormone that acts to increase blood pressure by constricting blood vessels.

As a woman's ovaries continue to fail to produce estrogen, the hypothalamus and the pituitary become overstimulated. Both a surplus of reproductive hormones and extra norepinephrine and other brain chemicals are produced. It appears that this overstimulation of the hypothalamus, rather than the lack of estrogen itself, is responsible for the hot flash, rapid heartbeat, and other vasomotor (blood vessel control) symptoms. Women who return their estrogen levels to near normal by taking hormone replacement therapy find that the frequency and severity of hot flashes diminishes.

If overstimulation of the hypothalamus, triggered by a lack of estrogen, is the cause of hot flashes, why don't all menopausal women experience them? Again, the fault may be with the hypothalamus. According to menopause expert Lila Nachtigall, M.D., in her book, *Estrogen*, scientists now believe some women are more susceptible than others to hot flashes because they lack an appropriate number of estrogen receptors. The fewer estrogen receptors the hypothalamus has, the more estrogen is required in the bloodstream to "turn off" the gland's activity.

As you'll learn in Chapter Six, there are several ways to manage hot flashes, even if you decide not to take HRT. For most women, hot flashes tend to decrease gradually in frequency and finally end within about three to five years, once the body has adjusted to its altered hormonal state.

SLEEP DISTURBANCES

Insomnia, or the inability to sleep, is second only to hot flashes as the symptom that first brings women entering the climacteric to their physicians. The trouble can occur in any part of the sleep cycle: some women have difficulty falling asleep, others wake up frequently during the night, and still others find themselves wide awake very early in the morning, long before their normal rising time.

For some women, the cause of their sleep disturbances are night episodes of a hot flash. Commonly known as night sweats, these unpleasant events often leave women soaked with sweat, shivering, and unable to fall back to sleep. Not all cases of insomnia in menopausal women can be traced to night sweats, however. The brain waves that control our sleep patterns, set by the hypothalamus, are also sensitive to the same overstimulation experienced by our temperature control system during menopause. When the hypothalamus works overtime in a vain attempt to produce enough GnRH to stimulate a follicle to ripen, our sleep may be disturbed by the erratic signals it sends.

Keep in mind, however, that sleep patterns naturally change as we age. The older we get, the less sleep we tend to need. Most infants, for instance, sleep more than fourteen to sixteen hours per day while adults usually require less than eight hours, and the elderly may get by on just four or five hours. If you find yourself sleeping fewer hours but feeling rested, chances are you have nothing to worry about. However, if you are sleeping less than five or six hours a night and are constantly exhausted, see your doctor.

Please note: although insomnia is a common symptom, many perimenopausal find themselves sleeping far *more* than usual. If you are sleeping more than ten hours a night and still do not feel completely rested, you could be suffering from depression or another illness. Consider seeing your doctor.

DERMATOLOGICAL CHANGES

Your skin is the largest organ in your body and, like all other organs and tissues, it changes as you age. Indeed, the signs of wear and tear are most visible on this, our only organ totally exposed to the environment. Both men and women experience the wrinkles, dryness, and diminished suppleness that affects the skin as they age. For women, however, this aging process appears to be accelerated by the loss of estrogen, which plays an important role in maintaining the health of the skin.

Your skin is made up of two major layers, the epidermis and the dermis. The main structural components of the dermis are protein fibers known as collagen, which depend to a large degree on the presence of estrogen. With the loss of estrogen at menopause, the amount of collagen decreases, causing the skin to pucker and wrinkle and hair follicles to weaken.

The skin is made up of three major layers: the epidermis, the skin's surface layer; the dermis, the middle layer; and the bottom layer made up of fatty tissue and muscle. Age and lack of estrogen affect each layer in a slightly different way. The epidermis, the skin's surface layer, constantly replaces itself as cells from below move to the surface while the surface cells die and flake off. The older we get, the thinner the epidermis becomes and the less often epidermal cells replenish themselves. In addition, as estrogen, which helps the epidermis stay moist and supple by stimulating water retention and oil lubrication, becomes less abundant, the skin tends to dry out and become taut.

By far, the most fundamental changes occur within the dermis, the middle and most substantial layer of the skin. Within the dermis are elastin fibers, blood vessels, hair follicles, sweat and oil glands, and nerve cells. Surrounding this tissue and comprising 97 percent of the dermis is a substance called collagen. Collagen, a protein that depends to a large degree on estrogen for its production, is an important component not only of the skin, but of connective tissue throughout the body, including bone, tendons, and ligaments. It is the amount of collagen in your dermis that is largely responsible for the elasticity, thickness, and tone of your complexion.

Like the cells of the epidermis, collagen is constantly being destroyed and replaced with healthy, new cells. As we age, however, collagen cells die at a greater rate than new ones are produced. Thus, the skin loses some of its elasticity and density and develops wrinkles as the tissue begins to fold in upon itself. Without estrogen, this breakdown of collagen occurs far more quickly than usual.

The bottom layer of the dermis, made up of fatty tissue and muscle, lends the skin thickness and elasticity as well. As you may remember, the distribution of fat throughout our bodies depends to some degree on the actions of the sex hormones: women tend to have an extra layer of fatty tissue throughout the body and even more fat in the hips and thighs. When the balance between estrogen and androgens begins to change during menopause, the fat layer beneath the skin tends to shrink and pucker—another cause of wrinkles.

It should be stated here that although estrogen, or the lack of it, does play an important role in the way our skin ages, it is hardly the only culprit. Two external factors—the sun and cigarette smoke—share equal responsibility. Both sap our skin of essential moisture. At the same time, cigarette smoke constricts the blood vessels, depriving the skin of oxygen while the sun destroys oil-producing glands as well as collagen. In addition, lack of exercise, a poor diet, insufficient fluid intake, and rapid weight losses and gains all contribute to the aging of our skin.

Directly related to age-related skin changes are shifts in the pattern of hair growth. Some women lose hair from all over their bodies at this time, others find hair growing where it had never appeared before. These variations occur for two reasons, both of them involving the unsettled hormonal state. First, the root of each hair—called a hair follicle—is located within the dermis. Surrounding the follicles and giving them support is tissue made up largely of collagen, which depends at least in part on estrogen for its health. As collagen levels diminish, the follicles become weak and hair falls out more easily. And, like other body cells, the hair follicles tend to replenish themselves less often and less quickly the older we get.

Just when some women find the hair on their heads falling out, however, they notice small growths of hair sprouting on their faces, backs, and chests for the first time. This occurs because androgens—male hormones—now play a greater role in our bodies than ever before. Without sufficient estrogen to oppose their action, androgens may cause hair to grow in a more typically male pattern. Hormone replacement therapy, described in Chapter Four, will help reverse some of the effects of aging on the skin and hair, and in Chapter Six you'll learn how best to take care of your hair and skin, before, during, and after menopause, so that the loss of estrogen need not take such a heavy toll.

FORMICATION

One of the most peculiar and frightening sensations described by menopausal women is formication: the feeling that insects are crawling over the skin. In fact, the word formication is derived from the Latin meaning "ant action." If you've ever had this experience, rest assured that you are not going mad and that you're not alone. About 15 to 20 percent of menopausal women experience formication at least once. Numbness, "pins and needles" and tingling sensations are also common. Like formication, they are vasomotor symptoms similar to hot flashes in that they are probably caused by an overstimulation of the blood vessels by the hypothalamus.

VAGINAL ATROPHY

Just like your skin, your vagina changes in many ways with age and loss of estrogen. In fact, vaginal tissue is more dependent on estrogen than any other part of the body. The vagina is made up of three layers: an internal mucous membrane lining responsible for providing lubrication and elasticity; a layer of connective tissue filled with tiny veins that fill with blood during sexual arousal, and a muscular layer that expands and contracts.

As estrogen levels fall, the mucous membrane tends to become thinner and less supple. This thinning may cause irritation, itchiness, and even bleeding that can lead to recurrent vaginal infections. After menopause, there is also a measurable decrease in the quantity and quality of vaginal secretions. Not only does the vagina become drier, but the lubrication secreted tends to be less acidic, which leaves the vagina open to yeast and bacteria that would have been neutralized by the previously high acid content of the secretions. The size of the vagina decreases as well, becoming shorter and narrower. Muscle tone also lessens, leaving the vaginal passage feeling slack and loose.

The external genitalia, called the vulva, also change with the loss of estrogen. The folds of skin called the labia and the area where the pubic hair grows, called the mons pubis, are designed to protect the clitoris and the vagina. As we age, we tend to lose pubic hair from the mons pubis and fatty tissue from the labia. This often results in a decrease in sensitivity to sexual stimulation.

The combination of these vaginal changes is called *vaginal atrophy*. As with other menopausal symptoms, the presence and severity of vaginal atrophy varies from woman to woman. It usually begins to occur about three to five years following the last menstrual period, although women whose ovaries are surgically removed may experience vaginal atrophy much more quickly due to the sudden and sharp decrease in estrogen production.

An unfortunate side effect of vaginal atrophy is the havoc it plays with a woman's sex life. Many women find that vaginal atrophy causes sexual intercourse to become so painful that they and their partners would rather avoid sex altogether. (See "Sex Drive Changes" below.) Luckily, treatment with estrogen, in the form of creams or pills, usually restores vaginal tissue quickly. Other self-help tips, covered in Chapter Six, may alleviate the problems as well.

BEST BET!

The term "use or lose it," as crude as it may sound, holds some truth when it comes to sex and the older woman. Studies show that vaginal symptoms of menopause are not as pronounced in women who have frequent intercourse and/or orgasms (defined as intercourse three or more times a month and orgasm at least once a week) as in celibate women.

URINARY TRACT DISTURBANCES

Located adjacent to the vagina and equally sensitive to estrogen are the organs of the female urinary tract. The urethra (the tube that carries urine from the bladder to the outside) and the bladder (a sac that acts as a reservoir for urine before it is expelled from the body) are both susceptible to similar atrophy: they become weak, thin, and more prone to infections and dysfunction. A woman afflicted with urinary atrophy may experience one or more of the following symptoms: dysuria, a burning sensation upon urination; urinary frequency, the need to urinate more often due to the thinness of the lower bladder wall; and urinary urgency, the strong desire to urinate and the inability to hold urine. Bladder infections also occur more frequently after menopause because the tissue is more fragile and thus more susceptible to infection.

SEX DRIVE CHANGES

For many women, sexuality becomes a major issue as they pass from fertility through the menopause. However, as is true for every other menopausal symptom, each woman will find herself reacting to sex in a uniquely individual way. One woman may find herself less interested in sex than before, while another discovers herself intrigued by as yet untapped sensual pleasures.

If you are passing through menopause and find yourself less interested in sex than you were before, the reason for your reticence could be physical: as described above, loss of estrogen often causes dryness and thinning of vaginal tissue, which may result in painful intercourse—a certain turn-off for both women and their partners. A loss of libido may be hormonally related: not only do the ovaries fail to produce female hormones following menopause, but they cease their output of testosterone—the male hormone linked to the female sex drive—as well. Another physical side-effect of aging is that it takes longer for both women and men to become aroused and to reach orgasm as they age. If communication is poor between partners, this change in the sexual routine may be, at least at first, a bit frustrating and embarrassing.

In addition to the physical reasons for a decline in libido are the many psychological barriers some older women feel lie between them and an active sex life. Many women feel less attractive to their partners as they age—no surprise in a society that worships the young and slender. Others lose their life partners to death or divorce around the time of menopause and are unable or unwilling to explore new sexual relationships.

The other side of sex and the menopausal woman is that many people find that the sex drive *improves* with age. Released from worries about pregnancy and birth control, some women find themselves feeling more confident and adventurous. By this time, too, the children have usually left home and women generally have more time to pamper themselves and their partners. Once any physical barriers to pleasurable sexual intercourse have been treated—by hormone replacement or even sex therapy—most postmenopausal women find themselves enjoying sex as much or more than before.

EMOTIONAL CHANGES

In addition to the physical symptoms of menopause, many women also find themselves feeling anxious, depressed, and emotionally erratic during this period. Like many other symptoms, these emotional changes have both a physical and psychological basis. First, the emotions are affected by the hypothalamus, the same part of the brain that controls your menstrual cycle. When the hypothalamus becomes overstimulated as your reproductive hormonal levels begin to decline, you may well become anxious, depressed, and irritable, at least until your hormonal levels stabilize.

At the same time, it is important to realize that external forces may be playing an equal part in your depression or anxiety. As you reach the age of menopause, you may encounter major shifts in your personal life. If you have children, they may well be on their way to independence, leaving you feeling a sense of loss. If you are childless, the realization that you *will* *never* bear children may upset you, even if it is a choice with which you're usually quite secure. If you're a career woman, you may be facing an impending retirement that leaves you feeling uncertain about your own self-worth. Your marriage may be undergoing stress and strain at this time, too, as your husband approaches retirement or passes through his own midlife crisis.

One of the largest hurdles you may have to face is the way today's society glorifies youth and fertility over the wisdom and sensuality of age. Developing enough self-confidence to ignore or overcome this cultural bias is no easy chore for most of us. The most important fact to remember is that what you are feeling is perfectly natural and you need only look to the more than 1.5 million women who pass through menopause every year for support. Read Chapter Six for tips on how to lift yourself up and out of the middle aged blues.

THE IMPORTANCE OF ATTITUDE

We've come a long way since doctors—mostly male doctors—were able to pass off our complaints about menopause with a condescending, "It's all in your head, dear." Indeed, the symptoms and side-effects described above have a very real physiological basis and cannot be avoided simply by ignoring them or by thinking positively.

HOT FLASH!
The Power of Positive Thinking

According to the Healthy Women Study, conducted at the University of Pittsburgh School of Medicine and presented at the 1991 Annual Meeting of the Psychosomatic Society, women who expected that learning the facts about menopause and maintaining a good attitude would help them have an easier time of it, did indeed experience lower levels of depression and fewer symptoms than women with pessimistic outlooks.

However, there does appear to be at least some connection between attitude and symptomology. Women who have a positive outlook on menopause, and about aging in general, appear to suffer fewer and less severe symptoms than do women who fear or loathe the idea of passing through this transition. A 1991 study conducted at the New England Research Institute and published as part of the Massachusetts Women's Health Study involved interviews with 2,565 women. Results showed that the majority of women who reported negative feelings about the cessation of menses felt worse—physically and emotionally—than did their peers with a more positive attitude.

For many women, the myths described in Chapter One only feed their fears about menopause and therefore make the experience more difficult and painful than it need be. Simply by reading this book, you've taken a big step forward: by learning about what menopause really means to your body and to your future, you're allowing yourself a chance to prepare for the physical and emotional changes in a realistic way.

Keep in mind that each and every woman experiences menopause in her own unique way. Some of us will pass through the transition to infertility easily, others may need some medical or psychological help. Without doubt, however, the years we have lived have begun to take their toll, particularly on two of the hardest working systems of the body: the cardiovascular system and our skeletal system. In the next chapter, you'll learn about the increased risks for heart attacks and osteoporosis among postmenopausal women and how to protect yourself from developing these all too common afflictions.

CHAPTER 3

> ## LONG-TERM COMPLICATIONS:
> ## OSTEOPOROSIS AND
> ## CARDIOVASCULAR DISEASE

Just about 150 years ago, a woman living in the United States could expect to die at or before the age of forty-one years. Today, thanks to improved medical technology and general knowledge about health care, most of us will live almost thirty-five years longer than our foremothers. However, in order to live those "extra" years of life with health and vigor, women must take special precautions against two of the most debilitating—and often lethal—complications of aging: osteoporosis and cardiovascular disease.

Until menopause, neither condition poses much of a problem among most women. Once our supply of estrogen is gone, however, both our bones and our blood vessels become more vulnerable to irreversible damage. Because some women are at greater risk than others of developing cardiovascular disease or osteoporosis, it is essential that we all learn what factors in our own lives may promote the development of these two deadly diseases.

OSTEOPOROSIS: OUR SILENT ENEMY

One of the most discouraging images of aging is the woman so crippled by the ravages of osteoporosis that she carries the dreaded "dowager's hump": bent from the waist, with her spine crushed to create a hump at about shoulder height, a woman with severe osteoporosis may lose as many as seven or eight inches of height to this progressive disease. In addition to the vertebrae of the spine, her wrists, forearms, and hips are also vulnerable; these bones may become so brittle that even a relatively minor fall or blow could cause them to snap in two.

Although to a young woman, a broken bone may seem no more than a bit painful and inconvenient, to an older woman who requires longer bouts of bed rest to heal, such an injury may be fatal. Over time, a completely sedentary body is susceptible to pneumonia as well as to pulmonary emoblism, a blockage of a blood vessel in the lung that causes pneumonia-like symptoms. Blood clots in the lung and in the extremities may also travel to the brain and heart, causing strokes and heart attacks. In fact, during the early 1970s, surveys revealed that as many as 10 to 15 percent of women who suffered a hip fracture died within four months of the fracture. Although new studies are now being conducted to confirm these statistics, morbidity rates for hip fractures are equally distressing today: osteoporosis is associated with approximately forty thousand deaths among women every year.

Osteoporosis affects at least half of all American women over the age of sixty. Its symptoms are usually so subtle as to be undetectable. The first sign that the disease has taken hold is often a bone fracture of the wrist, hip, or vertebra. In fact, osteoporosis involves a long process of bone degeneration that may start as early as thirty to forty years before the first signs appear. It progresses most after menopause, when bone loss among affected women may occur at a rate of 3 to 5 percent a year. At that rate, they will have lost more than 40 percent of their bone mass by the time they are eighty years old.

The term osteoporosis comes from the Greek *osteo* (bone) and *porus* (pore or passage). With osteoporosis, your bones become too weak to support the body. It occurs because your bones do not receive adequate nourishment to grow and renew themselves nor do they efficiently metabolize the nutrients they do receive.

Although we tend to think of bone as solid material, it is actually living tissue enriched by blood vessels that travel through it. Bone consists of two major layers of cells: the smooth outer surface tissue known as cortical bone and a spongy, meshlike material made up mostly of collagen, the protein-based connective tissue that also is a major component of skin tissue. When collagen is hardened by the mineral calcium, it forms a network of solid tissue called trabeculae.

With osteoporosis, bone loss occurs at a more rapid rate in trabecular bone than in cortical bone. While both trabecular and cortical bone are found throughout the body, their proportions vary from bone to bone. The vertebrae of the spine and the ends of the long bones of the arms and legs, for instance, contain more trabecular bone than other areas of the skeleton and are thus more prone to breaking and cracking when osteoporosis is present.

Like most other body tissue, bone cells are constantly dying and being replaced by new cells. The process of bone regeneration, or remodeling, consists of two distinct stages. During the resorption stage, special cells called osteoclasts dissolve some bone tissue, which creates a small cavity on the bone surface. During the formation stage, another type of cells, called osteoblasts, take nutrients from the bloodstream to fill the cavities.

The balance between osteoclasts and osteoblasts changes during your life. As an infant and teenager, you have many more osteoblasts than osteoclasts, and hence are able to build bone tissue easily. During your twenties, thirties, and forties, an absolute balance between osteoblasts and osteoclasts exits; you neither gain nor lose bone mass. As you age, however, the number of osteoblasts decreases while the number of osteoclasts remains about the same; therefore, more bone is destroyed than is able to be replaced.

THE CALCIUM CONNECTION

The primary nutrient contained in bone is calcium, a metallic element responsible for giving bones their strength and density. Calcium is not only important to the health and strength of bones, it is also essential to the proper functioning of many other parts of the body, including muscles, nerves, endocrine and exocrine glands, and blood cells.

Although calcium is only one factor in bone maintenance, it is an important one. Unlike some substances, such as cholesterol, our body does not produce any of its own calcium. To meet our daily needs, then, we must eat foods rich in calcium or take calcium supplements. Otherwise, we risk losing bone mass; once lost, bone is almost impossible to regenerate.

After calcium is consumed into the stomach, it is absorbed through the intestinal wall into the bloodstream and carried to sites in the body requiring the mineral. Vitamin D, a fat-soluble vitamin we receive from both vegetables and sunlight, allows this absorption to take place; a deficiency of vitamin D, either from a poor diet or lack of sunlight, leads to decalcified, brittle bones, a condition known as rickets.

Once in the bloodstream, more than 99 percent of the body's calcium eventually winds up being stored in bone tissue. Through an elaborate system of hormonal checks and balances, an adequate amount of calcium is circulating in the bloodstream at all times: if your body does not receive enough calcium from your diet every day to meet all its needs, it will take calcium from your bones to make up the difference. The sex hormones estrogen (in women) and testosterone (in men) appear to help protect bones from being "robbed" of calcium by other parts of the body.

A certain amount of bone loss is to be expected as a natural part of aging. First of all, a chronic lack of sufficient calcium—which affects millions of people—will rob bones of their needed strength over time. Second, like all other human tissue, bone cells are replenished less often as we get older. When menopause occurs, and the hormones that would protect us dramatically decline, this mild bone loss may develop into the chronic, debilitating condition known as osteoporosis.

Although men do not undergo the equivalent of menopause, they too experience some acceleration in bone loss as they age. This loss rarely causes osteoporosis, largely because men generally have heavier, denser bones than do women. In addition, testosterone production declines very gradually and to a much lesser degree than estrogen declines in women; the available testosterone provides men with several more years of protection against bone loss than women who do not replace estrogen. Indeed, during the five years following their last periods, women lose bone mass twice as quickly as men of the same age.

Although no one knows exactly what role sex hormones play in bone metabolism, it appears that estrogen actually stimulates the production of another hormone, known as calcitonin. Calcitonin helps facilitate the uptake of calcium from the blood into the bone by the osteoclast cells and, at the same time, inhibits the loss of calcium from the bone by the osteoblasts. In addition, estrogen helps produce and maintain collagen, an important component of bone; as in skin, the collagen content of bone decreases in direct relationship to the decrease in estrogen level during menopause.

THE RAVAGES OF OSTEOPOROSIS

As stated above, the porous trabecular bone, which is especially prevalent in the spine and in the long bones of the arms and legs, is most affected by osteoporosis. The holes within the trabecular bone widen, until the bone is eventually unable to support the surrounding cortical shell (see Figure 2, below). A slight fall or blow is all that is needed to fracture a bone beset by osteoporosis.

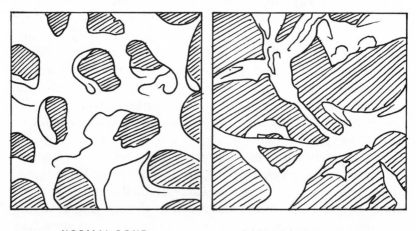

NORMAL BONE   OSTEOPOROTIC BONE

FIGURE 2 Osteoporotic bone. The drawing on the left shows the internal structure of healthy bone. Note the thick bridges of trabeculae (hardened collagen and protein) between the pores. On the right, note the bone weakened by osteoporosis. The pores are much larger and the trabeculae are thin and fragile.

The bones in the spinal column, called vertebrae, are often the first to become injured. About one out of every four women has at least one vertebral fracture by the time she reaches the age of sixty; by the age of seventy-five, more than 50 percent succumb to some degree of spinal osteoporosis. When vertebrae fracture, they collapse, one upon the other, often without causing any pain (see Figure 3, below). In fact, a woman may first discover that she has osteoporosis in her spine while being x-rayed for an unrelated reason. Or, even more likely, she will visit her doctor after making the startling discovery that she is shrinking in height. Indeed, every time a vertebra collapses, a woman loses about an inch of height; depending on the severity and speed of osteoporosis, it is possible for a woman to lose several inches within just a few months.

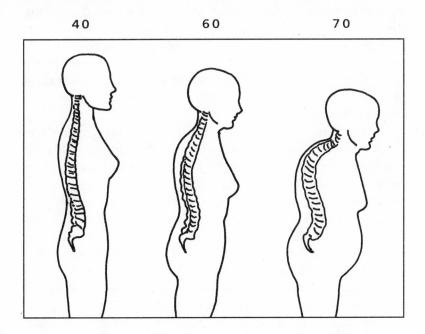

FIGURE 3   Postural changes in women with osteoporosis. The dreaded "dowager's hump" that results from osteoporosis develops gradually, over decades, as the bones of the spine weaken and collapse due to lack of calcium.

If many vertebrae collapse, her spinal column will gradually form an exaggerated curve, her rib cage will fall, and her stomach will protrude. As her body collapses upon itself, her internal organs are adversely affected: breathing may become labored as the lungs lose the room they need to expand and contract properly, a condition known as atelectasis; constipation often occurs because the intestines are unable to digest food properly; back and leg muscles may become strained trying to keep the misshapen body upright and mobile. As common as the condition may be, it remains one of the most physically—and emotionally—crippling side effects of the aging process. Not only is a woman with severe osteoporosis uncomfortable and, to some extent, immobilized, she is also frequently embarrassed or ashamed about her appearance.

Other common sites of fractures due to osteoporosis are the wrists and the hips. Many women break their wrist bone as they attempt to break a fall; it is only after they visit their doctors that they realize they are suffering from osteoporosis. Hip fractures are the most serious injuries suffered by women with osteoporosis. As mentioned above, many women are permanently disabled by the break; others succumb to complications that eventually kill them. In fact, hip fractures are the twelfth leading cause of death in the United States today.

It may surprise you to know that many women discover they suffer from osteoporosis during a visit to their dentists. Although poor gum care often takes the blame for tooth loss in the elderly, osteoporosis instead may be the culprit. The disease tends to thin out the jawbone, so that teeth have no firm base in which to anchor themselves. They eventually loosen and fall out. To add insult to injury, finding comfortable, snug-fitting dentures are almost impossible for the osteoporotic patient because the jaw-bone continues to change shape and shrink.

As stated at the beginning of this chapter, osteoporosis is a common disease, eventually affecting about 50 percent of all women after menopause. But what about the other 50 percent? Why don't their declining levels of estrogen affect their bones to the same degree? It appears that several factors, including heredity, lifelong calcium intake, and level of physical fitness all have an impact on your risks for developing osteoporosis.

RISK FACTORS FOR OSTEOPOROSIS

Gender

According to the National Osteoporosis Foundation, women are four times more likely than men to develop osteoporosis. As discussed, women both have thinner bones than men in general and suffer from a dramatic decline in estrogen—a substance that protects against bone loss—at menopause, while men's supply of testosterone is only gradually depleted.

Age

The older you are, the thinner your bones will probably be, largely because your body regenerates itself less efficiently as you age. In addition, many older people fail to exercise or eat the appropriate amount of calcium every day. However, the crippling effects of osteoporosis are *not* part of the normal aging process; osteoporosis is a disease that requires treatment and care.

Heredity

Women with a family history of osteoporosis are more likely to develop the disease.

Ethnicity

For reasons not yet fully understood, Caucasians of northern European descent, especially women with light eyes and fair skin, have the highest incidence of osteoporosis. It is epidemic among Japanese and other Asian women as well. African-Americans, Hispanics, and women of Mediterranean ancestry appear to be most immune; the incidence of hip fractures is about twice as high among white women as in black women. Jewish women fall in the middle of the range.

Physical build

Because petite women with small bone structures have less bone mass to start with, they are at a higher risk of osteoporosis than large-boned women. A slender build also increases risk; fatty tissue converts adrenal hormones to estrogen, so very thin women have lower levels of estrogen. Heavier women are at less

risk. The stress of the excess weight on their skeletons stimulates their bones to grow bigger. (Please note, however, that the
health risks of obesity, including diabetes, heart disease, and
stroke, far outweigh its protection against osteoporosis.)

Premature menopause

After menopause, the rate at which bone is lost more than
quadruples among most women. Women who have an abrupt
and early menopause because of hysterectomy or chemotherapy
develop osteoporosis at an earlier age and with more pronounced
bone loss than women who undergo a later, natural menopause.

Sedentary lifestyle

In addition to nutrition, exercise plays an important role in
bone metabolism. Like muscles, bones respond to exercise by
growing stronger and larger. Exercise stimulates the production
of certain hormones, including estrogen, as well as increases
the amount of blood flow throughout the body. Weight-bearing
exercises that cause muscles to work against the force of gravity, such as walking, stair-climbing, running, and tennis, are
particularly effective in helping to prevent bone loss.

Cigarette smoking

Women who smoke lose bone mass more quickly and more
severely than their smoke-free counterparts, largely because
smoking appears to affect both estrogen production and the
way estrogen is metabolized. (And, as discussed in Chapter
Two, smokers tend to undergo menopause from five to ten
years earlier than nonsmokers. The longer one is without estrogen, the more bone loss occurs.)

Alcohol and caffeine

In large amounts, both of these substances accelerate bone
loss by interfering with calcium and vitamin D metabolism in
the liver. The more alcohol and caffeine you consume, the
greater your chances of developing osteoporosis. (Moderate
alcohol intake appears to help prevent cardiovascular disease,
however. See Chapter Seven.)

Calcium deficiency

Many women, especially those with an aversion to dairy products, may have a chronic calcium deficiency without knowing it. According to the National Dairy Council, more than three quarters of American women over thirty-five fall far short of the 800 milligrams (mg) Recommended Dietary Allowance set by the National Academy of Sciences. Furthermore, both the National Institutes of Health and the National Osteoporosis Foundation recommend that postmenopausal women not on hormone replacement therapy receive a daily allowance of at least 1,500 mg of calcium, almost *twice* the level set by the National Academy of Sciences. The problem of calcium depletion may be compounded among women who have had several children and breastfed their babies without taking adequate dietary calcium during pregnancy and lactation.

Diseases

Certain diseases and conditions seem to predispose an individual to osteoporosis. These include rheumatoid arthritis, diabetes mellitus, chronic kidney disease, and disorders of the thyroid, parathyroid, or adrenal glands.

Drugs

Certain medications, taken at high dosages over long periods of time, may influence the development of osteoporosis. These drugs include thyroid replacement drugs, heparin (an anticoagulant), some cortisone preparations (such as prednisone), and the antibiotic tetracycline, among others. Some diuretics used to treat high blood pressure may increase the risks, while others, particularly thiazide diuretics, may actually have a positive effect on bone. If you suffer from hypertension and are at risk of osteoporosis, talk to your doctor about the right medication for you.

Pregnancy

Childbearing, which promotes the production of estrogen and progesterone, appears to have a protective effect on the bones, provided the expectant mother is well-nourished; however, if she does not take in enough dietary calcium, the calcium for the baby's nutritional needs will come from the mother's bones. Breastfeeding when the mother is not well-nourished also depletes calcium.

DIAGNOSING, PREVENTING, AND REVERSING OSTEOPOROSIS

After reading about the risk factors listed above, do you feel you're at risk of developing osteoporosis? If so, speak to your doctor about your concerns. If the condition runs in your family or if you've experienced bone fractures, your doctor may decide to perform one or more medical tests, called absorptiometry or densitometry, that measure bone mass in various sites in the body. (For more information, see Appendix I.)

Unfortunately, once bone mass is lost, there is little you can do to restore it. But you can prevent further loss from occurring and, with hard work, perhaps replace at least some of what has been lost. To do so involves instituting a program of lifestyle changes—and perhaps medication—that can prevent future bone loss and fractures.

Eat a calcium rich diet

Calcium is important throughout a woman's life. Although from ages eighteen to thirty-five bones no longer grow, they continue to increase in density. If a woman eats enough calcium during her early adult years, she can build up her bones to their maximum potential. In Chapter Seven, you'll learn how to increase your dietary calcium, even if you don't like to eat dairy products. You'll also discover the pros and cons of calcium supplements and how to choose the most efficient supplement available.

Exercise daily

This is the only preventative measure that can actually add mass to bones—provided you also receive sufficient calcium from your diet. The most effective bone-building exercises are those that stress the long bones of the body (arms and legs), such as jogging, walking, bicycling, and aerobics. (If you've already suffered bone loss, particularly from the spine, talk to your doctor about choosing exercises that will not add further stress.)

Stop smoking

Cigarette smoking is one of the most damaging habits known to woman or man. Not only does smoking increase risks of cancer and cardiovascular disease, it also affects menopause and osteoporosis.

Hormone replacement therapy (HRT)

The American Medical Association, the National Institutes of Health, and the Federal Drug Administration all agree that replacing estrogen and progesterone in women who have undergone menopause significantly reduces their risks of developing osteoporosis. According to the National Osteoporosis Foundation, women who choose to go on hormone replacement therapy suffer from 50 to 70 percent of hip fractures compared with women who do not. However, there are risks as well as benefits associated with HRT. (Read Chapter 4 for more information.)

Other treatment

A relatively new drug called etidronate, marketed under the name of Didronel, is one of the best bone-sparing drugs available for women unable to take estrogen. It works by suppressing the action of osteoclasts, the cells that dissolve bone tissue, as well as helping the bones absorb calcium. Paired with calcium and vitamin D supplements, Didronel has proven to be a very safe and effective medication for menopausal women suffering from osteoporosis.

Another drug, recently approved by the FDA, is calcitonin, a hormone made in the thyroid gland. Calcitonin decreases bone resorption, or the breakdown of bone, by acting directly on osteoclasts, the cells on the surface of cells instrumental in rebuilding bone matter. However, calcitonin, which is administered by injection, should be used only in cases of severe calcitonin deficiency and only if estrogen therapy is contraindicated. Another substance under investigation is sodium fluoride, which also works primarily on vertebral bone. However, fluoride treatment has not yet been approved by the FDA, mainly because of its side effects, including anemia, joint inflammation, and stomach upsets.

If you feel you are at risk for osteoporosis, it's important to eliminate as many risk factors and add as many healthy habits to your life as possible. Luckily, most of the changes you'll make will also help you protect yourself against another leading health problem for women after menopause: cardiovascular disease.

CARDIOVASCULAR DISEASE: OUR SILENT AND GROWING ENEMY

Although we tend to think of cardiovascular disease—specifically strokes and coronary artery disease—as a "man's problem," women, especially as they pass the age of menopause, are indeed at risk. In fact, cardiovascular disease accounts for more than ten times the deaths among women than breast cancer every year.

It remains true, however, that women suffer from less cardiovascular disease than men—at least until menopause. At the age of fifty and younger, a man is six times more likely to die from a heart attack than a woman of the same age. Within ten years after menopause, however, the female advantage against heart attacks has been lost.

It is unclear exactly why this marked disparity exists, but researchers believe that the female hormones, estrogen and progesterone, play an important role in protecting women from the ravages of atherosclerosis, otherwise known as hardening of the arteries, which is a main risk factor of hypertension and heart disease. Testosterone, on the other hand, has no such protective effect; in fact, the male sex hormone may actually promote the development of atherosclerosis. When women pass the age of menopause and their hormone levels decrease, their rates of high blood pressure, atherosclerosis, and heart disease catch up and even surpass those of men.

The good news about cardiovascular disease is that there are proven ways of both preventing the conditions associated with it from ever developing and of reversing the disease even after some damage to the heart and blood vessels has already occurred. First, however, it's important to learn how a healthy heart and circulatory system work and what may be putting you at risk of cardiovascular disease.

YOU AND YOUR CIRCULATORY SYSTEM

In order to live, each cell of the body must have a steady supply of oxygen and other nutrients as well as a way to eliminate the waste products it produces. The human circulatory system that transports these nutrients and wastes consists of two main components: the blood itself and the vessels that carry the fluid. The heart, a sac of specialized muscle tissue, lies at the center of this system. Essentially a sophisticated pump, the heart rhythmically contracts, about seventy-two times a minute, to force the blood out through the vessels and then back to the heart.

The average adult has about eleven pints of blood, which the heart pumps through the body. Every time the heart beats, it sends two to three ounces of blood from its pumping chamber (the left ventricle) into the largest artery (the aorta). The large arteries that supply blood to the head, internal organs, and the arms and legs stem from the aorta; these large arteries then branch into smaller and smaller vessels, the smallest being the arterioles and capillaries. On the way back to the heart, the blood travels through veins and their smaller subset, venules. Remarkably, it only takes about a minute for a drop of blood to make its way through the more than seventy thousand miles of blood vessels in the average human body.

Most diseases of the blood vessels, including those that cause heart attacks and strokes, can be traced back to the condition known as atherosclerosis. Atherosclerosis occurs when the walls of the blood vessels become thickened by an accumulation of material, including fats and lipids. Cholesterol, a fatty substance that is both consumed in the diet and produced by the body, is a major factor in the development of atherosclerosis.

High blood pressure is one of the by-products of the atherosclerotic process. When an artery narrows, blood pressure goes up as the heart pumps harder and the arteries constrict more strenuously to push the blood through. Slowly but surely, the arteries affected by atherosclerosis become so narrowed that blood can no longer pass through at all. If enough plaque accumulates, blood flow through the artery becomes totally blocked, causing a stroke or a heart attack. Atherosclerosis also results in increased blood clotting, which may also cause heart attacks and strokes.

A heart attack is the common name for a myocardial infarction, which occurs when one of the vessels leading to the heart becomes so clogged that heart tissue dies due to lack of oxygen. When arteries feeding the brain become blocked, a stroke results. In this case, the brain cells once fed by the blocked vessel are destroyed by the lack of oxygen.

THE CHOLESTEROL-ESTROGEN CONNECTION

Cholesterol is now the great American dietary enemy and largely with good reason. Too much of a certain kind of cholesterol can, indeed, damage the health of our cardiovascular system. But many people are unaware that some amount of cholesterol is essential for the human body to function properly. It is used to manufacture hormones and vitamin D, for instance, and is present in virtually all body tissue. When too much cholesterol is circulating in the blood, however, the disease of atherosclerosis may result.

Cholesterol travels through the bloodstream by combining with lipids (fatty substances) and certain proteins; when combined these substances are called lipoproteins. It is the relationship between different kinds of lipoproteins that determines the amount of cholesterol circulating in the bloodstream. Low-density lipoproteins (LDL) carry about two thirds of circulating cholesterol to the cells; this is often the "fat" we speak of when referring to the plaques that build up and cause atherosclerosis. High-density lipoproteins (HDL), on the other hand, carry cholesterol *away* from the cells (and blood vessel walls) to the liver, where it is eliminated from the body.

At birth, the human body contains about half of its cholesterol in the form of HDLs, but because the typical American diet is so high in cholesterol, we tend to replace HDLs with LDLs as we grow older. When you have more LDLs than HDLs, your body is transporting more cholesterol *into* the bloodstream, which increases your risk for atherosclerosis and heart disease. If there is more LDL in your blood, you are said to have more "bad" cholesterol, since more of this fatty substance stays in the bloodstream than is eliminated.

BEST BET!
Have Your Cholesterol Checked Regularly

A common myth about high cholesterol is that only overweight people are susceptible. In fact, anyone, especially someone with a family history of high cholesterol or diabetes, can be affected.

Have your cholesterol level measured soon. The National Cholesterol Education Program, sponsored by the National Institutes of Health, recommends that desirable total blood cholesterol should be below 200 mg/dl. A reading between 200 to 239 is borderline, and any reading over 240 mg/dl is considered high. LDL cholesterol categories are as follows: less than 130 mg/dl is desirable; 130 to 159 mg/dl is borderline high; and over 160 mg/dl is high. HDL levels for women should range from 37 to 42.

Most cases of high cholesterol can be controlled by diet and exercise. (See Chapters Seven and Eight for more details.)

Estrogen, it appears, helps maintain a healthy balance between LDL and HDL levels during a woman's fertile years. The exact mechanism by which it does so is as yet poorly understood, but several studies show that when estrogen is withdrawn, through natural menopause or hysterectomy, the amount of "bad" cholesterol increases dramatically. When postmenopausal women take hormone replacement therapy, on the other hand, both their cholesterol levels and their risks for heart attack and stroke decrease dramatically. (More on hormone replacement therapy and heart disease in Chapter Four.)

RISK FACTORS FOR CARDIOVASCULAR DISEASE

The impact of the loss of estrogen upon a woman's cardiovascular system is highly individual. Some women completely escape the devastating effects of atherosclerosis after they lose estrogen, while others succumb rather quickly. Clearly, estrogen alone is not the only culprit for the majority of women who suffer from cardiovascular disease. Indeed, there is a long list of both hereditary and lifestyle factors that combine to put a woman at risk.

Your Cardiovascular Self-Test

Answer each question yes or no.

___ **Are you over 50?**

Although aging itself does not cause cardiovascular disease, many diseases that promote its development, such as diabetes mellitus and hypertension, also tend to develop later in life, as do the effects of life-long bad habits, such as smoking, excessive alcohol consumption, or overeating and obesity.

___ **Do strokes or heart attacks run in your family?**

Along with other traits like eye color and height, your parents may have passed on to you certain physical characteristics that put you at risk for cardiovascular disease.

___ **Do you have high blood pressure?**

High blood pressure, which is both a cardiovascular disease itself and a risk factor for other types of vessel disease, including coronary artery disease and stroke, is epidemic in this country, affecting more than thirty million Americans. Over a period of years, high blood pressure can damage the arteries throughout the body so that the artery walls become thickened and stiff—a condition called arteriosclerosis. Hypertension also damages the walls of the vessels in such a way as to promote the formation of fatty plaques, the cause of atherosclerosis. There are many causes of hypertension and, fortunately, many quite effective treatments. However, like osteoporosis, it is often a silent killer: many women suffer from hypertension without ever being aware of it. If hypertension runs in your family, be sure to have your blood pressure monitored by your physician, especially as you get older. (See Appendix I for more information about blood pressure monitoring.)

___ **Do you suffer from diabetes mellitus?**

Diabetes mellitus, or the inability to metabolize carbohydrates, is another prevalent disease in modern America, affecting more than fourteen million people. A person with diabetes either does not produce enough of the hormone insulin, which is largely responsible for regulating the body's metabolism, or is unable to use the insulin properly. Diabetic patients have a much higher incidence of cardiovascular disease, including hypertension and stroke, than do nondiabetic patients. Experts feel that this is due in part to the fact that people with diabetes have a much higher level of fat in the bloodstream than do those with normal sugar metabolisms. The famous Framingham Study, a four-decade study in which five thousand patients from Framingham, Massachusetts were monitored for cardiovascular disease, 80 percent of the deaths among women with diabetes were due to cardiovascular disease.

___ **Do you smoke cigarettes?**

If you smoke, you dramatically raise the risks of developing cardiovascular disease, whether or not you've reached menopause. The Surgeon General reported in 1989 that more than two hundred fifty thousand deaths from heart attacks and stroke are directly related to smoking. Cigarette smoking raises the amount of fats and cholesterol circulating in the bloodstream, which form plaque on artery walls. In fact, cigarette smoking has been shown to raise the level of low-density lipoproteins by as much as 10 percent. Another ingredient of cigarette smoke, carbon dioxide, helps the process along by damaging the cells that form the inner linings of arterial walls, making them more susceptible to plaque buildup.

___ **Are you overweight?**

According to a 1990 report by the Framingham Study Group, obesity is a major cardiovascular risk factor. Even ten extra pounds puts an incredible burden on the heart and blood vessels; for each pound of excess weight, the heart is forced to pump blood through an additional several hundred extra miles of blood vessels a day. Overweight people also tend to eat too much fat and cholesterol, which contributes to atherosclerosis. As many women pass the age of menopause, the tendency to gain weight increases, largely due to a more sedentary lifestyle. However, this weight gain will put you at much greater risk for cardiovascular disease, especially when you no longer have estrogen to protect you.

____ **Do you exercise regularly?**

It is becoming more and more clear with every study that a vigorous, regular exercise routine may help to prevent cardiovascular disease. Exercise helps improve the health of the entire circulatory system by distributing the blood more evenly to all blood vessels. Vigorous exercise also appears to lower the level of LDLs (the "bad" cholesterol) while raising HDL levels. Another good reason that exercise helps prevent heart and vessel disease is that it burns calories and increases our metabolism, helping to prevent us from gaining weight. As we've discussed, obesity is a major risk factor for cardiovascular disease, especially among postmenopausal women.

How many of these risk factors apply to you? Even if you've checked off a bunch, don't despair. Although you are powerless to change your gender, your age, and the time you experience menopause, there is plenty you can do through proper diet, exercise, and other lifestyle changes to protect yourself from cardiovascular disease. In fact, if you suffer from diabetes or hypertension, the same lifestyle changes you make to protect your heart will help you keep these chronic conditions under better control.

In addition to lifestyle changes, which will be covered in Chapters Seven and Eight, many women at risk for both cardiovascular disease and osteoporosis may benefit from hormone replacement therapy (HRT) after menopause. There are risks as well as benefits from HRT, however, and it's important for you to weigh all your options before deciding whether or not to replace the estrogen and progesterone no longer manufactured by your ovaries. Chapter Four will help you make that decision.

CHAPTER 4

THE ESTROGEN QUESTION

To take estrogen or not to take estrogen? To prescribe estrogen or not to prescribe estrogen? Among both patients and physicians, the relative risks and benefits of hormone replacement therapy (HRT) form the heart of one of the hottest medical controversies of the day. Available to women whose ovaries no longer produce sex hormones, HRT attempts to replace estrogen and progesterone so that the female body will continue to function much as it had before ovarian failure.

By taking HRT, menopausal women hope to avoid not only the discomfort of hot flashes, night sweats, and other symptoms, but also prevent the development of certain long-term complications of hormonal loss, including osteoporosis and heart disease. Today, most researchers agree that HRT effectively accomplishes these goals for most women. However, as with any medical treatment, HRT involves some risks as well as benefits. Whether or not the risks outweigh the benefits—or vice versa—is still under intense debate.

Just twenty to thirty years ago, most physicians routinely prescribed estrogen to their menopausal patients; in the early 1970s, estrogen was the fifth most commonly prescribed drug in the United States. But during the mid-1970s, several studies reported a marked increase in endometrial cancer among women on long-term estrogen therapy. In fact, cancer rates were up to thirteen times greater in women taking estrogen for five years or more than in women who did not take the hormone.

At the same time, another estrogen-based drug, called diethylstilbestrol, or DES, made the headlines. Administered during the 1950s and 1960s to prevent miscarriages in pregnant women, DES was found to have had serious side effects, including profound birth defects in the children of women who took it.

In addition, studies concerning the side effects of the birth control pill also deterred physicians and patients from estrogen replacement. Oral contraceptives, which used relatively high dosages of estrogen and progesterone, were linked to an increase in strokes, heart attacks, and abnormal blood clotting. Moreover, several studies in the 1980s showed a disturbing, although as yet unconfirmed, link between long-term estrogen use and breast cancer. However, what many women do not know is that in the twenty years since the first reports about cancer and estrogen were issued, great strides have been made in developing safe and effective hormone therapy. The birth control pill of the 1990s, for instance, is more effective and safer for more women than ever before. By reducing the amount of female hormones contained in each dose, manufacturers of oral contraceptives have been able to reduce the risks of heart and circulatory disorders in most women.

Using a similar approach, scientists have been able to make hormone therapy safer and more effective for menopausal women, too. Today, HRT involves a combination of estrogen—in much lower dosages than in the past—and progesterone that appears to significantly reduce the risk of endometrial and other cancers. In addition, study after study confirms the fact that estrogen has a protective effect against osteoporosis and cardiovascular disease in postmenopausal women.

Nevertheless, resistance to HRT remains strong—in fact, just 15 percent of all menopausal women in the United States take hormone replacement therapy today—partly because women have very real, and realistic, fears about potential side effects. Although cancer and vascular disease risks from estrogen therapy are much lower than they were twenty years ago, they still exist. Indeed, for women with certain medical preconditions—such as breast cancer or prior history of abnormal blood clotting—the risks may outweigh the benefits.

Some women resist taking hormones not only for medical reasons, but also because they feel that menopause is a natural transition—not a "disease" that needs medical intervention.

On the 1992 publication of her book about menopause, *The Change*, feminist Germaine Greer told *Newsweek* magazine, "You can't try to postpone the inevitable. The whole thing about women is that they change. We are the changeable sex." In fact, claims Greer, the promotion of hormone replacement therapy is merely another way of telling a woman that her only worth stems from staying young and beautiful. "All around you, the message is that once you're old, you are worthless..."

A *Boston Globe* newspaper column by Linda Weltner on August 23, 1992, cites another theory about the current focus on HRT, posed by Alice Rossi of the Social and Demographic Research Institute at the University of Massachusetts/Boston. Rossi proposes that doctors and pharmaceutical companies have more to gain from HRT—in terms of fees and profits—than women do from its therapeutic effects. Millions upon millions of our foremothers went through menopause without the need for drugs, claim proponents of this theory, and it is only to feed the greed of the medical industry that HRT exists to the extent it does today.

On the other side of the HRT coin are those women who believe that replacing estrogen is a healthy choice, both medically and emotionally. Unlike most medications, HRT is not *adding* foreign substances to the body, but is rather *replacing* essential substances that your body can no longer produce naturally, much like insulin in the body of a diabetic. Furthermore, our foremothers did not "need" HRT because many of them died before or just after menopause and thus did not live for years with the debilitating symptoms and side effects of a body deficient in estrogen. Indeed, because a woman now lives more than a third of her life after menopause, many physicians and their patients feel that estrogen is essential to protect the body from osteoporosis and heart disease.

Without question, HRT is not for everyone. In the end, the decision about HRT rests with each individual woman and her physician. A woman's past medical history, her symptoms during perimenopause, her special risks for osteoporosis and heart disease, her cultural and sociological slant on the matter—as well as her gynecologist's medical opinion—all come into play.

What every woman owes to herself, however, is to make certain that her decision is an informed one. Although it goes far beyond the scope of this book to outline all the risks and benefits as they may apply to you, if you read this chapter carefully, you'll at least know the right questions to ask your doctor when the time comes for you to decide about HRT.

THE RIGHT COMBINATION

Until the beginning of the 1980s, most women who decided to take hormones to relieve their menopausal symptoms were given doses of estrogen only. The current trend is to oppose estrogen with progesterone, the hormone the ovaries would naturally produce during the second half of the menstrual cycle. An estrogen-progesterone combination therapy allows a woman's body to experience a monthly cycle similar to the one she had before menopause. As stated above, such a combination has been found to significantly reduce the risks of endometrial cancer associated with unopposed estrogen.

Before we delve into how the new combination estrogen-progesterone therapy affects the risks and benefits of HRT for you, let's discuss what HRT actually entails.

TYPES OF ESTROGEN

As you may remember from Chapter One, estrogen is a term used to describe a broad category of related female sex hormones. In humans, there are three principal natural estrogens: estradiol, estrone, and estriol, with estradiol being the most potent and active form. Estrogen therapy preparations use varying amounts of these estrogens alone or in combination.

Estrogen exists in many dosages and forms. Synthetic estrogens are produced in the laboratory using artificial, petroleum-based chemicals. Natural estrogens are identical to those found naturally in the body and are derived from animal sources. In general, the synthetic estrogens are more potent than the natural preparations—in fact, they are used chiefly in the manufacture of the birth control pill, which requires high dosages of estrogen in order to suppress ovulation—and thus have more severe side effects. Almost all women using HRT to relieve menopausal symptoms take natural estrogen.

Of the dozen or so different natural estrogen preparations, the most commonly prescribed brand is a conjugated equine estrogen known as Premarin. Conjugated estrogens are a mixture of naturally occurring estrogens derived from the urine of pregnant mares (hence its name: *Pre* [for pregnant]—*mar* [for mare]—*in* [for urine]). Premarin comes in both pill form and in a vaginal cream. Another common estrogen preparation is estrone, a weak form of estrogen produced both by the ovaries and through the conversion of androgens by fat cells. Estrone also comes in pill and cream forms under the brand name Ogen. Estradiol, a more potent form of estrogen, is the main constituent of the pills marketed under the brand name Estrace. Estradiol is also available in a transdermal patch under the brand name Estraderm.

Oral estrogen

Estrogen comes in pill form, usually taken once a day by mouth. Once swallowed, it is absorbed by the intestines and sent through the bloodstream to the liver. The liver then metabolizes the estrogen to estrone, the form of estrogen that works on the tissues in the body. As it travels through the liver circulation, estrogen stimulates other proteins and substances produced in the organ. Some of these substances are beneficial to the body, such as HDL (the "good cholesterol") which helps to lower the risk of atherosclerosis. Other substances produced by the liver after estrogen stimulation produce negative results, such as angiotensinogen, which elevates blood pressure in some women.

Although oral estrogen is the most commonly used and easiest to administer, it is not for everyone. Because naturally occurring estrogens are insoluble in water, their absorption from the stomach or intestines is limited; therefore, some women do not absorb enough of the hormone to receive therapeutic results. Other women have liver disease, gallbladder disease, or blood clotting disorders that would be exacerbated by estrogen stimulation of the liver. (See below under "Risks of HRT.")

Fortunately, there are several other ways to administer estrogen that bypass digestion and liver metabolism altogether, including:

Vaginal estrogen cream

Hormones applied directly to vaginal tissue provide relief to women who suffer from localized vaginal discomfort, such as dryness or itchiness, or urinary tract infections. Although some of the hormone eventually reaches other parts of the body through the blood stream, vaginal cream is not effective for relieving other common symptoms and side effects of menopause, including hot flashes, night sweats, or osteoporosis and heart disease. On the other hand, some estrogen from the cream *does* circulate in the body; therefore, this method is inappropriate for women who are not supposed to take estrogen.

Transdermal patch

The most recent—and welcome—breakthrough in estrogen therapy is the skin patch, which is marketed in the United States under the brand name Estraderm. It works like this: a patch dispensing the required dose of estrogen is applied to the skin (usually on the hip, thigh, or abdomen) once or twice a week. Estrogen is released from the patch directly into the bloodstream (thereby bypassing the liver) in a steady, constant dosage. For most women, the effect on menopausal symptoms and long-term side effects is equal or greater than that found with oral estrogen. In fact, a small study conducted in Milan, Italy and published in the journal *Minerva Endocrinologica* in January, 1989, showed that women who use skin patches gain quicker control of hot flashes than those who use oral preparations.

On the other hand, some women find that the patch causes the skin beneath it to become itchy and sore; this can often be resolved by placing the patch on tougher skin, such as on the buttocks or the back. Others find they need more estrogen than they did when they were taking oral preparations. In addition, because the patch allows the estrogen to avoid the liver, the hormone no longer stimulates the production of HDL cholesterol. It does, however, work to lower LDL (the "bad cholesterol") levels, thereby producing a better overall lipid profile in most women.

For women who do not like to take pills every day, or for whom oral estrogen is contraindicated, the transdermal patch appears to be a godsend. However, as with other estrogen preparations, women who use the patch must also take progesterone, which comes in pill form (see below), for a prescribed number of days every month in order to simulate a regular hormonal cycle.

Injection

In rare cases, estrogen is injected in the muscle tissue of women unable to take estrogen by mouth. This method has largely been supplanted by the transdermal patch.

Estrogen pellets, gels, and tablets

Although not yet approved by the FDA, these methods also bypass the liver and are considered by some women to be easier to use and just as effective as oral estrogen. One such method involves implanting a capsule of the hormone beneath the skin. The pellet will then release a low but steady dose of estrogen into the bloodstream every day from six to twelve months.

In Europe, some women use an estrogen gel that is rubbed into the skin of the abdomen and is thus absorbed into the bloodstream. This form of estrogen tends to be less reliable than others because a woman may inadvertently vary the amount she applies to the skin from day to day. Yet another mode of application not yet available in this country is buccal estrogen, a tablet that dissolves in the mouth and is absorbed through the mucous membranes into the bloodstream. These tablets appear to be especially effective in controlling hot flashes.

TYPES OF PROGESTERONE

Most women who take estrogen therapy must also take progesterone concurrently. As described in Chapter One, progesterone becomes active in the second half of the menstrual cycle; if an egg is fertilized, progesterone helps to further stimulate the growth and nourishment of the egg and the uterine lining, called the endometrium. If an egg is not fertilized, the progesterone breaks down the endometrium, which is then flushed out of the body during the menstrual period. This flushing out process cleans the uterine lining, leaving it healthy and ready to receive a fertilized egg during the appropriate time in the next cycle.

Without progesterone, the endometrium would receive what is known as *unopposed estrogen* stimulation. The continued growth of the endometrium results in what is known as hyperplasia, which is considered a precancerous condition. Many scientists believe that this buildup of endometrial cells is responsible for the increased risk of endometrial cancer associated with estrogen therapy in menopausal women.

Progesterone is part of a class of hormones known as progestins. Like estrogen, progestins are either derived from natural, animal sources or produced synthetically; synthetic progestins tend to be stronger than natural progestins and, like estrogen, are used most often as a component of the oral contraceptive. There are several different types of progestins that are used as part of HRT. Medroxyprogesterone acetate, known by the brand names Provera, Amen, and Curretabs among others, are the most commonly prescribed progestins. Megesterol acetate, or Megace, and 17a hydroxyprogesterone caproate, or Delalutin, are also prescribed. All progestins come in pills to be taken orally, although some can be formed into suppositories for women who are unable to take oral progestin.

THE HRT REGIMEN

How much estrogen and progestin is required to treat menopausal symptoms? That figure varies slightly from woman to woman and depends on how much estrogen she normally produced during her fertile years. If you have not yet passed through menopause, your gynecologist may decide to test your blood levels for FSH/LH (follicle-stimulating and luteinizing hormones) to see how much of these hormones you produce naturally. In addition, the blood levels of estradiol, a form of estrogen, may also be tested. Estradiol levels can range anywhere from seventy to three hundred, depending on when in your menstrual cycle the test is performed. Most gynecologists prefer testing at the beginning of the cycle, when the follicle is producing high levels of estrogen.

If your doctor knows the level of estrogen normally circulating in your blood, he or she will be better able to prescribe the best dosage of estrogen for you after menopause. If you don't have that information available to you, you'll probably find you need to try several different dosages of estrogen to find the one that suits you best.

Generally speaking, however, most gynecologists would agree that when it comes to hormones, less is best. The more estrogen you take, the greater your risk of developing uncomfortable and potentially dangerous side effects. Lila Nachtigall, M.D., associate professor of obstetrics and gynecology at New York University School of Medicine and director of the Women's Wellness Center at New York University Medical Center, suggests that 1.25 mg of conjugated estrogen per day should be the upper limit for most women on HRT; taking less than .625 mg every day will probably not provide either symptomatic relief or long-term protection against osteoporosis and heart disease.

The amount and dosage of progestin you should take depends to a large degree on what type of hormone replacement regimen you and your doctor decide is right for you.

Cyclic regimen

Most women today choose to take HRT in such a way as to mimic the menstrual cycle. If you decide to go this route, you'll take oral estrogen (probably about .625 mg per day) for about twelve days, then estrogen and progestin (in 5 to 10 mg per day dosages) together for about thirteen days. After twenty-five days, you'll stop taking both pills. At this point, you will probably experience withdrawal bleeding from the vagina, though not as heavily as during a normal period.

If you opt for the transdermal patch, you'll find that it comes in two doses: 0.05 mg—which is about equal to a dosage of .3 mg to .625 mg of Premarin—and 0.10 mg which is about equal to between .9 and 1.25 mg of the oral estrogen preparation. Each patch is effective for about three days; therefore you'll be changing the patch twice a week. Progestin dosages and schedules remain the same as with oral estrogen.

Combined continuous therapy

A new approach to estrogen-progestin therapy involves taking *both* an estrogen and a low dose of progestin (usually 2.5 mg) every day of the month. This method protects the endometrium from constant estrogen stimulation while eliminating withdrawal bleeding. Since most women look forward to the day when they can stop worrying about their monthly periods, this type of HRT regimen is sure to become more popular. The major complaint among women on combined continuous therapy is breakthrough bleeding (spotting), although by fine-tuning hormone dosages this problem is usually eliminated within six months or so.

Continuous progestin therapy

Some women, because they suffer from breast cancer, uterine cancer, or have severe fibrocystic breast disease, are unable to take estrogen in any dose. Progestin taken alone has been found to help alleviate hot flashes as well as provide protection against osteoporosis by improving calcium metabolism. However, progestin will not improve symptoms of vaginal atrophy, such as dryness or itchiness, and may actually promote atherosclerosis.

Other forms of menopausal therapy

In addition to progestin, other medical alternatives exist for those who cannot take estrogen. Although none of them work as quickly or as effectively as estrogen, they may relieve some menopausal symptoms. One such drug is clonidine, a medication often used to treat hypertension. Clonidine, manufactured under the brand name of Catapres, is known as a central brain stem agonist: it works to decrease the activity of the sympathetic nervous system, which diminishes the tightness of the blood vessels and thus alleviates the occurrence of hot flashes. However, clonidine may cause unpleasant side effects, such as dryness of the mouth, fatigue, irritability, dizziness, and headaches in some women.

Bellegral (phenobarbital) and other sedatives may relieve hot flashes and other vasomotor symptoms. Tranquilizers, such as Valium and Librium, may help some women who are troubled by anxiety, irritability, and mood swings during menopause. However, since these drugs may be addictive and may cause serious side effects, including depression, they should be used only under a physician's careful supervision and only as a last resort.

THE SIDE EFFECTS OF HRT

Although most women find that their menopausal symptoms almost completely disappear with HRT, their relief does not usually come without a price. Indeed, many hormone users experience side effects from their medication. Some of these symptoms disappear within six months or so after therapy is initiated; those that do not can usually be treated effectively through diet and exercise (see Chapter Six for more details). All of them are reversible once treatment is stopped.

Fluid retention

The most common side effect of HRT, affecting more than 50 percent of menopausal women on estrogen, fluid retention occurs because estrogen increases salt retention, and excess salt in the bloodstream causes more water to be retained by the body. Some physicians will prescribe a diuretic to relieve this symptom and/or recommend making dietary changes such as reducing your intake of salt and caffeine.

Breast swelling and tenderness

Called mastalgia, this condition is caused not by estrogen itself but by the effects of progestin on estrogen in the breast tissue, which may cause fluid retention and breast swelling.

Abdominal cramps

As you may remember, during a normal menstrual cycle, estrogen promotes the buildup of the endometrium (the lining of the uterus) and progesterone causes the endometrium to break down. Cramping may occur during the later phase through the hormonal stimulation derived by HRT as well as natural menstruation.

Headaches

Another side effect of estrogen is an increase in migraines, especially in women prone to these headaches. It appears that the brain, along with other body tissue, may retain more fluid when estrogen is present. Some women have such severe migraines with HRT that they decide to forgo the treatment rather than suffer with them.

Weight gain

About 25 percent of women on estrogen therapy report putting on weight, especially when they first start therapy. Fluid retention is once again the most likely culprit and most women find their weight stabilizes after several months to a year on HRT. However, as stated in Chapter One, menopause comes at time when many women decrease the amount of exercise they perform just when their bodies' metabolic rates slow down. In other words, estrogen is only part of the problem when it comes to gaining weight after menopause. (See Chapters Seven and Eight for more details.)

Nausea

As described above, estrogen taken in pill form must first be digested and absorbed by the intestines before reaching the bloodstream. Some women who take oral estrogen become nauseous during this phase. If this symptom does not improve after a few weeks, use of the transdermal patch or vaginal cream may be indicated.

THE IMPORTANCE OF MONITORING

How long should a woman remain on HRT? Many doctors now agree that in order to be effective against osteoporosis and heart disease, hormones should be continued for as long as a woman lives. However, and this is a *big* however, a woman on HRT must be willing to be carefully monitored and supervised by her physician for as long as she remains on hormones.

Why is monitoring so important? First of all, as discussed above, most women on HRT need to fine-tune their dosages and methods of application before finding the right regimen:

one that will relieve symptoms and promote bone retention and cardiovascular health without causing side effects. In fact, you can expect about a two to three month period during which your body adjusts to the hormones. After that time, if you are still experiencing side effects, you may be on too high or too low a dosage.

If the dose of estrogen is too high, your breasts may feel tender, you may notice an increase in vaginal discharge because your cervix is secreting more lubrication and you may be retaining fluid. If the dose of estrogen is too low, your menopausal symptoms will not be alleviated. At this point, your doctor will probably decide to perform a blood test to monitor the level of estradiol in your bloodstream. If your pre-menopausal estradiol level is known, your doctor will try to match the level produced with HRT, which should eliminate symptoms. If not, you may need to try several different dosages in order to find one that alleviates your symptoms without causing side effects.

Second, HRT is not without its risks. Estrogen affects the way many different organs function, including the liver, the heart, the uterus, the ovaries, and the breasts. In order to make sure that estrogen does not damage tissue, several tests should be performed on at least a yearly basis:

- Pelvic and breast examinations
- Mammogram
- Pap smear

In addition, a biopsy of your endometrium is necessary whenever you have unexplained vaginal bleeding or if endometrial cancer runs in your family. Cholesterol levels should be checked regularly with a blood test as should heart function with an electrocardiogram. A bone density test to determine the presence of osteoporosis is also recommended for all women as they enter the climacteric, but especially for those who are at high risk. (See Appendix I for more information about medical tests.)

Now that you know what HRT really entails, you're in a better position to judge the risks and benefits of hormone therapy as they may apply to you. Let's start with the risks.

THE RISKS OF HRT

Endometrial cancer

The most well-publicized risk associated with the use of HRT is cancer of the lining of the uterus, called the endometrium. Today, endometrial cancer ranks third among the most common cancers in women with an estimated annual incidence in the range of 39,000 to 42,000 cases. In 1987 alone, the National Cancer Institute estimated there were 2,900 deaths from endometrial cancer and 35,000 new cases developed in the United States.

Cancer, of which there are more than one hundred different types, involves the abnormal proliferation of cells. The cause of most cancers is largely unknown, although some substances—called carcinogens—are known to increase the risk of cancer. Tobacco; certain chemicals such as nickel, asbestos, and other industrial agents; excessive alcohol intake; and exposure to radiation are just a few known carcinogens. In some individuals exposed to these substances, cancer develops.

In addition, a tendency to develop some types of cancer may be inherited and other conditions, such as diabetes, obesity, high cholesterol, and other diseases, may also increase an individual's cancer risk. Endometrial cancer, for example, has several risk factors associated with it. Women who have a family history of the disease are at higher risk than those who do not, as are those with hypertension and those who have never carried a pregnancy to full term. Obesity appears to be one of the greatest risk factors in the incidence of cancer—about 73 percent of women diagnosed with endometrial cancer are more than 20 percent over their proper weight.

Estrogen, which has been linked to a rise in endometrial cancer, is not a carcinogen. It may, however, cause a buildup of the endometrium called hyperplasia. In some women with other risk factors for endometrial cancer, hyperplasia may develop into endometrial cancer if allowed to continue to build up without a periodic sloughing off of tissue every month. Estrogen may also accelerate the growth of a cancer already present in the uterus (and in certain types of breast cancer), making screening for uterine cancer a must for all candidates for HRT. Hyperplasia and endometrial cancer may occur more often in women prone to those conditions when estrogen is taken unopposed. However, women who take progestins with estrogen appear to be at *no increased risk* of developing endometrial cancer compared with postmenopausal women who do not take estrogen.

Breast cancer

Approximately 10 percent of women in the United States will develop breast cancer during their lifetime. The incidence increases with age: it occurs in 27 per 100,000 women aged 30 to 34; in 102 per 100,000 women aged 65 to 74, and in 422 per 100,000 women aged 70 to 74. For the year 1991, the National Institutes of Health have estimated that in the United States 175,000 new cases developed and approximately 44,500 deaths were caused by breast cancer.

As with endometrial cancer, your risk of developing postmenopausal breast cancer depends on a wide variety of risk factors, including family history of breast cancer or fibrocystic breast disease, obesity, and perhaps a diet high in fat. In addition, it appears that the longer you menstruate, the greater your risks of developing breast cancer. Therefore, if you were younger than twelve years of age when you first got your period, you run up to four times the risk of someone who starts to menstruate at the age of thirteen or older. If you are fifty-five or older when you pass through menopause, you have twice the risk of developing breast cancer than women who have their last periods at the age of forty-five.

Estrogen therapy may increase the risk of breast cancer in certain women, but the link between the two is still highly controversial. The tissue in a woman's breasts is as sensitive to estrogen as is the tissue that lines her uterus. Although there is not a periodic building up and shedding of breast tissue, certain women experience abnormal cell growth and the formation of benign cysts with estrogen therapy. In some women at risk for breast cancer, these formations may later develop into breast cancer.

In addition, there appear to be certain breast cancers that are more susceptible than others to estrogen stimulation. These cancers are called estrogen-dependent cancers, and they generally occur more often in postmenopausal women. Under no circumstances should estrogen therapy be given to women with estrogen-dependent breast cancer. However, in those cancers that are *not* estrogen-dependent, the addition of estrogen has been found to actually *decrease* the size of tumors, especially when it is combined with progestin.

Most physicians and scientists now agree that women who take low dosages of estrogen combined with regular cycles of progestin run no increased risk of breast cancer. In fact, an analysis of all recent literature concerning breast cancer and HRT was performed at the Department of Preventive Medicine, Vanderbilt University School of Medicine in Nashville, Tennessee and published in the January 1991 issue of *Archives of Internal Medicine*. This analysis confirmed that menopausal therapy consisting of .625 mg or less of conjugated estrogens does not increase breast cancer risks.

How does one explain the few studies that show an increase in breast cancer in women who take estrogen? Some evidence suggests that because women who take HRT are more likely to be under close medical supervision breast cancer screenings are done more often and more thoroughly than in women who do not visit their gynecologists as often. Therefore, breast cancers that would have developed with or without estrogen are being detected earlier and more often in women on HRT. Indeed, breast tumors diagnosed in women who use estrogen are smaller and carry a better prognosis than those diagnosed in women who are not on hormone replacement therapy.

Thromboembolic disease

Otherwise known as blood clots, thrombi and emboli are a major cause of heart attacks and strokes. In high dosages, including those found in birth control pills, estrogen may stimulate the production of some clotting factors produced by the liver. On the other hand, conjugated estrogens, especially in the low dosages found in most HRT regimens, do not appear to affect the liver clotting proteins or the tendency to clot among women who take them. Only a woman with a pronounced history of thromboembolic disease runs any increased risk of developing clots while on HRT.

Gallbladder and liver disease

The gallbladder is the sac located beneath the liver that stores the bile produced by the liver; bile is used to digest fatty substances after they enter the small intestine. Estrogen has a tendency to increase the cholesterol fraction of the bile, which may result in the formation of gallstones—hard masses of bile pigments, cholesterol, and calcium. The incidence of gallstones in postmenopausal women using HRT is about 2.5 times greater than in women not using hormones. Gallstones may be painful and may require surgery to remove.

In rare cases, women taking oral contraceptives may develop a cancerous tumor of the liver. Thus far, however, these tumors have not been reported in women using estrogen as part of HRT for menopause. However, women with previous histories of liver disease should be followed closely, especially at the beginning of the regimen.

Taken together, the risks of HRT may seem overwhelming. Why put yourself at *any* increased risk of cancer, stroke, heart attack, or liver disease just to prevent a few hot flashes? Yet all the evidence seems to point to the fact that—except for a small percentage of women who are particularly prone to certain conditions because of a genetic tendency or past medical history—HRT provides medical benefits that far outweigh the risks. Indeed, rather than putting themselves in danger, most women appear to derive some protection *against* endometrial and breast cancer with estrogen-progesterone therapy.

In 1983, the *Journal of the American Medical Association* published the results of a six-year study of estrogen use and all causes of mortality among about twenty-three hundred women across the country. The study found that estrogen users had a lower incidence of any kind of death than nonusers. Those women who had had their ovaries removed and took HRT had only 12 percent the incidence of death experienced by their counterparts who took no hormones. Estrogen users with intact ovaries had less than half the risk of death from all causes than nonestrogen users after menopause.

As discussed in Chapter Three and further delineated below, two diseases—osteoporosis and heart disease—are far more common and deadly than either breast or endometrial cancer among women. (About one woman in one thousand per year is diagnosed with endometrial cancer, compared with fourteen in one thousand per year with cardiovascular disease.) Many physicians feel that the protective effects of estrogen and progesterone on bones and blood vessels add several years of health to the majority of postmenopausal women. Therefore, unless you know you are more prone to certain conditions affected by estrogen stimulation, refraining from HRT may put you at far greater risk for more common and equally life-threatening conditions.

Moreover, menopause can cause symptoms that are just plain annoying and uncomfortable. Hot flashes, rapid aging of the skin, vaginal changes, and mood swings are hardly life-threatening, but they are certainly troublesome. Described in depth in Chapter Two, these side effects from the loss of estrogen may all be quickly and effectively diminished with HRT.

THE BENEFITS OF HRT

Strong and healthy bones

Osteoporosis affects more than 50 percent of post-menopausal women; preventing this progressive and debilitating disease from developing remains the single most pressing reason to take HRT. In fact, estrogen-progesterone treatment appears to be the *only* established measure that reduces the frequency of fractures due to osteoporosis after menopause. Not even high dosages of calcium can help a woman with osteoporosis from losing more bone mass unless estrogen is also present.

In addition, the longer a woman is without estrogen, the more brittle her bones become. Therefore, hormone replacement therapy to protect against osteoporosis is particularly important for women who go through premature menopause due to oophorectomies, chemotherapy, or other conditions that cause ovarian failure.

To be effective, HRT must be initiated as soon as possible after menopause and must continue for a considerable period of time, for at least five to ten years or for the rest of a woman's life if she shows no adverse reactions from the treatment. Sufficient calcium intake (from 1,000 to 1,500 mg per day) and weight-bearing exercise such as stair climbing, walking, or jogging will add to the protective benefits of HRT. In fact, exercise may restore bone mass in some women. (See Chapters Seven and Eight for more information about dieting and exercising to strengthen your bones.)

A strong and healthy cardiovascular system

Without question, the loss of estrogen has a profound effect on a woman's heart and blood vessels. According to the Framingham Study—an intensive, thirty year examination of risk factors for cardiovascular disease among approximately five thousand residents of a small Massachusetts city—postmenopausal women who did not take estrogen had more than double the incidence of cardiovascular disease as premenopausal women.

Although estrogen's role in cardiovascular health is well-documented, there is concern among the medical community that the addition of progesterone to the regimen—essential for protecting against endometrial and, perhaps, breast cancer—may reverse estrogen's beneficial effects. Indeed, many progestins promote atherosclerosis by causing a rise in the LDL-cholesterol level and a fall in the HDL-cholesterol level—just the opposite of estrogen's positive effects.

However, several studies show that the protection provided by estrogen usually overwhelms progesterone's negative effects. A 1990 study conducted at the George Washington University Medical Center and published in the February 1991 issue of *Obstetrics and Gynecology* showed that the addition of a progestin to estrogen therapy caused only a slight elevation in LDLs while allowing estrogen to continue to lower the amount of total circulating cholesterol, thereby promoting a generally more favorable overall lipid profile in women taking the hormones.

Normal vasomotor reactions (no more hot flashes!)

For most women, the relief of hot flashes—those rushes of heat and moisture that seem to come at the most inopportune moments—is the most significant benefit of HRT. Other vasomotor symptoms, including palpitations, dizziness, and numbness, are also relieved by the effect estrogen has on the hypothalamus—the hormone-producing gland responsible for many of our bodily functions, including blood pressure, sleep patterns, and, of course, the menstrual cycle.

Healthier and younger skin and hair

As discussed in Chapter Two, estrogen affects every layer of your skin, providing it with moisture, fullness, and elasticity. Without HRT after menopause, your skin may show the signs of aging far more quickly and dramatically than if you took hormones, becoming drier, thinner, and more prone to wrinkling. Within six months of taking HRT, however, most women find a more youthful luster and softness returning to their skin. Because estrogen stimulates water retention, skin also tends to plump up, which diminishes wrinkling. At the same time, hair follicles remain strong with estrogen, thereby helping to retain the hair's thickness and luster.

Supple vaginal tissue

Vaginal atrophy—the shrinking and drying of vaginal tissue due to lack of estrogen—is one of the most common and uncomfortable side effects of menopause. With HRT, especially in the form of vaginal estrogen creams, vaginal atrophy can be halted and reversed within four to six weeks. Hormonal therapy will also alleviate the increase in vaginal infections many women experience after menopause.

A healthy urinary tract

As you may remember from Chapter Two, the same kinds of changes that take place in the vagina also may occur in the urinary tract after menopause. Fortunately, urinary tract infections, stress incontinence, and irritable bladder syndrome are also relieved by HRT. Certain exercises that tighten the walls of the vagina and the urethra (called Kegel exercises) may also help keep your urinary tract functioning properly. (See Chapter Six for more details.)

A healthy sex life

Many women find that their sex lives remain active, or even improve, after menopause if they take HRT. Vaginal tissues remain supple and lubricated, while progesterone continues to stimulate the libido. In addition, with menopause comes freedom from pregnancy and birth control; many women find that this freedom translates into heightened libido and sexual response.

A healthy and energetic outlook

For many women, taking HRT means the end to the mood swings, irritability, and even bouts of depression that plagued them after menopause. Part of this "return to normalcy" no doubt derives from the fact that other debilitating and depressing symptoms that may come with the loss of hormones, such as vaginal atrophy, hot flashes, skin aging, and hair loss, improve with HRT. Obviously, a healthy sex life also goes a long way in brightening our moods.

The return of estrogen and progesterone also helps to stabilize the activity of the hypothalamus, which helps to control our emotions. In addition, there appears to be a connection between the estrogen-progesterone cycle and the release of beta-endorphins, the secretions from our central nervous system associated with the "runner's high" experienced by many athletes. A series of studies have shown that beta-endorphins rise and fall in response to the sex hormone cycle, and anything that reduces estrogen or progesterone levels also seriously limits the blood levels of endorphins. Returning hormone levels to normal, on the other hand, keeps those inspiring endorphins coming.

"To take estrogen or not to take estrogen?" After reading this chapter, do you feel in a better position to answer the question first posed at the beginning of this chapter? It is true that weighing the risks and benefits is often a confusing process, no matter how much information you have available to you.

In order to help you apply what you have just read to your own situation, we've devised the following "HRT Guide." Answer the questions to the best of your ability, then take the results with you the next time you visit your gynecologist.

Your HRT Guide

___ Does osteoporosis run in your family?

___ Are you fair skinned or small boned?

___ Do you have a family history of heart disease or atherosclerosis?

___ Were your ovaries removed or did your ovaries fail because of chemotherapy or another condition before you went through menopause?

___ Did you experience menopause before the age of 45?

___ Do you suffer from severe hot flashes, vaginal atrophy, loss of energy, or loss of libido?

The more questions you answered with a "yes," the more likely it is that HRT is more than just beneficial to you; it may be an essential ingredient for a long and healthy life—especially if you have gone through premature menopause. (Read more about hysterectomy and premature menopause in Chapter Five.)

Only if you suffer from certain conditions that may prevent you from taking hormones (see below) should you refrain from obtaining a prescription for HRT right away.

___ Do you have endometrial cancer or a family history of the disease?

___ Do you have unexplained vaginal bleeding?

___ Have you had breast cancer?

   ___ If so, was the cancer estrogen-dependent?

___ Is there a history of breast cancer in your family?

___ Do you suffer from liver disease?

If you answered yes to any of these questions, you and your

doctor may decide that the risk of causing or exacerbating diseases to which you are prone far outweighs the benefits you would receive from HRT. As discussed, estrogen acts on many different parts of the body, including the liver and breasts, in addition to the uterus and ovaries. Adding estrogen to the body may stimulate cancerous cells already present in these organs—though perhaps as yet undiscovered—to grow more rapidly. Any unexplained vaginal bleeding may indicate that the uterus has developed a cancerous tumor; until the cause of the bleeding is diagnosed, you should not risk estrogen therapy.

Keep in mind that not all women with breast cancer are ineligible for estrogen replacement. Most breast cancers that develop *after* menopause, for instance, are nonestrogen dependent; they will not be affected by estrogen and, in fact, may actually decrease in size with the addition of the hormone. Talk the matter over with your doctor.

If you answered "no" to the above questions, does this mean you are free to take HRT? In most cases, yes. On the other hand, there are some conditions that are exacerbated by HRT; although most of them are non-life-threatening, they do require special attention and monitoring. See if you suffer from any of these conditions.

Do you suffer from:
1) ___epilepsy?   5) ___hypertension?
2) ___uterine fibroids?   6) ___migraines?
3) ___heart or vessel disease? 7) ___endometriosis?
4) ___gallbladder disease?   8) ___fibrocystic breast disease?

1) In extremely rare cases, fluid retention—a common side effect of HRT—may cause epileptics to suffer an increased number of seizures. If you have epilepsy and decide to take HRT, you and your doctor should keep careful track of seizure activity.

2) Uterine fibroids are dense growths of tissue on or within the uterus; although noncancerous, they can grow to more than a foot in diameter. Hormones, especially estrogen, can stimulate fibroid growth. As fibroids may be painful, some women

choose to suffer the effects of menopause rather than risk stimulating fibroid growth with estrogen; others find they are able to manage only on low dosages. If fibroids continue to grow out of control, with or without HRT, your doctor may recommend a hysterectomy. (See Chapter Five for more details.)

3) Although in most cases, HRT works to protect your cardiovascular system from disease, in some cases of previously existing, serious heart or vessel disease, the addition of progesterone may cause just enough of an increase in the amount of "bad cholesterol" circulating in the bloodstream to warrant refraining from HRT therapy. Again, monitoring of your cardiovascular system through electrocardiograms, blood lipid profiles, and other tests further defined in Appendix I, may help your doctor devise a low enough progesterone dose to protect both your uterus and your heart.

4) As stated earlier in the chapter, the incidence of gallstones in postmenopausal women is about 2.5 times greater than in women not using hormones. If you have a history of gallstones, talk to your doctor before embarking on hormone replacement therapy.

5) Hypertension, or high blood pressure, is the most common cardiovascular disease in the United States, affecting an estimated sixty million people. There are many different types of hypertension, including rare cases caused by overstimulation of the liver tissue by estrogen. Because hypertension is easily and effectively treated with drug therapy, however, most physicians find that the benefits of estrogen on other parts of the cardiovascular system are well worth the need for additional medication.

6) Fluid retention in the brain may cause some people already prone to migraines to suffer more headaches. Fluid retention related to HRT often disappears after several weeks; if not, your doctor may be able to adjust the dosage of estrogen to relieve water retention.

7) Endometriosis is a disease in which cells of the uterine lining become displaced and attach themselves to other parts of the body, where they grow during the estrogen-progesterone cycle. Many premenopausal women who suffer from chronic

endometriosis require total hysterectomies, which entail the removal of the uterus, the fallopian tubes, and the ovaries. Then, when HRT is initiated, no endometrial cells are left to be stimulated by the hormones. In women with less severe symptoms, endometriosis usually disappears completely once the natural estrogen-progesterone cycle abates during menopause. Many of these women find that they can tolerate very low dosages of HRT to relieve menopausal symptoms without stimulating a recurrence of their disease.

8) As many as 40 to 60 percent of all women develop small, benign lumps—or fibroids—in their breasts. When these fibroids fill with fluid, they are known as cysts. If you have been diagnosed with fibrocystic breast disease, it means that you have a tendency to develop these harmless—although often painful and tender—fibroid cysts. Some studies show a correlation between fibrocystic breast disease and the eventual development of breast cancers; others show no such link.

Some cases of the disease can be treated through diet, by lowering fat and caffeine intake while increasing Vitamin E and Vitamin B complex. Since fluid retention may cause the breast tissue to swell and add pressure to the cysts, some physicians recommend that their patients take a diuretic about a week before the onset of their periods.

If you have fibrocystic breast disease and desire to go on HRT, you will have to be monitored carefully by your physician for two reasons. First, because estrogen may exacerbate fluid retention, you may require a particularly low dose of the hormone to avoid increased breast tenderness and pain. Second, the slight increased risk of breast cancer with HRT requires yearly breast exams; because cancerous tumors can be mistaken for cysts in manual exams, an annual mammogram is required as well.

After answering the questions in the "HRT Guide," do you feel HRT is right for you? Even if you're among the women who, for medical and/or personal reasons, decide not to take hormones after menopause, there are many other ways to relieve your symptoms and help protect yourself against long-term complications. (See Chapters Six, Seven, and Eight.)

In the meantime, it's important that we discuss what may occur if you go through premature menopause—before you pass the age of about forty—either due to total hysterectomy or to ovarian failure from chemotherapy or other conditions. Under what circumstances are hysterectomies really necessary? Do they always entail removal of the ovaries? Is menopause different for a woman who has her ovaries removed or whose ovarian cells are killed by chemotherapy or radiation? These and other important questions will be addressed in Chapter Five.

CHAPTER 5

PREMATURE MENOPAUSE AND HYSTERECTOMY

Although we tend to think of menopause as a natural transition that occurs about half to two thirds of the way through a woman's life, millions of women every year experience premature menopause—menopause that occurs ten or more years before the age of fifty-one. Women who pass through menopause early—for chemical, surgical, or natural reasons—deserve special attention because they often suffer from more abrupt and severe symptoms than women who experience natural menopause later in life.

Even those who pass through premature menopause easily must be extra-vigilant about their health as they grow older: the longer a woman is deprived of estrogen, the more brittle her bones and the more clogged her arteries may become, to say nothing of the long-term effect the loss of hormones may have on the condition of her skin or on her sex life due to estrogen-related changes to her vaginal tissue.

Who is most at risk for undergoing premature menopause? By far, the most common reason for premature menopause is the oophorectomy: the surgical removal of both ovaries as part of a hysterectomy to treat ovarian cancer or other cancers of the reproductive system, severe endometriosis, life-threatening infections, or to protect women from perceived risks of future cancer. As we'll discuss later in the chapter, the need for many hysterectomies and oophorectomies has been questioned in recent years; every woman should be aware of her options when it comes to deciding if this serious, life-altering surgery is necessary for her.

About 5 percent of all women inherit a tendency toward early menopause from their mothers and are born with thousands fewer eggs than most women. Others may have inherited an autoimmune disorder in which their own immune system destroys healthy ovarian cells for as yet unknown reasons. Although it takes place earlier than for most, the menopause these women experience generally occurs gradually, over several months or even years, and it is accompanied by the same range of symptoms seen in older women as they go through menopause. Other diseases that cause a hormonal imbalance may also result in amenorrhea (failure to menstruate) and, if persistent and incurable, early menopause.

Thousands of women every year pass through menopause in their forties, thirties, and twenties—even while still in their teens—because their ovaries are destroyed by chemotherapy or radiation therapy used to treat cancer. Designed to kill malignant cells, these treatments may also destroy healthy tissue, including ovarian cells that produce estrogen and progesterone. Although women with cancer of the female sex organs may expect to lose fertility to the disease and its treatment, women with cancer of the breast, lung, bone, brain, blood, or other tissue may be shocked to learn that menopause is often one of several side effects that results from treatment.

Radiation therapy, which consists of localized doses of gamma rays from nuclear sources, is not likely to harm tissue it does not affect directly; only women who take radiation for cancer located in or near the ovaries should expect to suffer long-term hormonal effects from it. Chemotherapy, on the other hand, travels through the bloodstream to the tumor it is meant to treat, often causing havoc along the way. Although many women find that chemotherapy is not nearly as devastating as they had expected, most do experience some nausea, anemia, and hair loss.

In addition, some chemotherapy patients learn that ovarian cells are among the healthy tissue destroyed by the drugs aimed at the malignancy. Even while fighting for their lives, these women are faced with menstrual irregularities, hot flashes, mood swings, and other symptoms of menopause that often come abruptly, intermittently, and quite unexpectedly. In some cases, ovarian function is irrevocably destroyed. Luckily, most women are able to take hormonal replacement therapy to correct the resulting imbalance.

A woman whose cancer treatment results in early menopause may need extra support from her friends and family over the issues of fertility loss and the common—if often unfair—link between menopause and old age made in our society. In addition, the symptoms and the long-term side effects associated with menopause may be both more severe and more complicated to treat than in women who go through a natural menopause. Already feeling out of control because she is facing a life-threatening disease, a woman who loses ovarian function at the same time may be especially troubled and may benefit from counseling and group support to help her cope.

HYSTERECTOMIES AND OOPHORECTOMIES

The statistics have made the headlines more than once during the past few years: nearly 50 percent of American women will have hysterectomies at some point during their lives. American women have hysterectomies five times more often than do their European counterparts; by the age of forty-two, more than 20 percent of American women have had a hysterectomy as compared with just 4 percent of European women. At approximately 650,000 per year, hysterectomy is the most frequent major operation performed on women in the United States today. More shocking is the fact that doctors themselves now admit that perhaps as many as 50 percent of these operations may be medically unnecessary.

Why are female sex organs taken out so often in the United States? The most cynical among us point to the fact that the operation is usually both simple and quite lucrative to the surgeons performing them—far more lucrative than the time-consuming office visits required to treat and monitor many diseases. Second, Americans physicians tend to perform surgery more often to treat all kinds of conditions—not only gynecological complaints—than do physicians in other countries.

Until recently, most doctors subscribed to the notion that female organs were more trouble than they were worth once the age of child-bearing had passed. In other words, once a woman no longer needed her uterus to carry a child or her ovaries to produce eggs, doctors felt that her increased risk of abnormal bleeding, cysts and fibroids, and cancer warranted the removal of these organs, almost as a matter of course.

Luckily, things are beginning to change. More and more doctors are beginning to recognize that the uterus and ovaries are indeed important to a woman's health even after menopause. The ovaries continue to produce a variety of hormones, including androgens. As you may remember from Chapter One, androgens are converted to estrogen by fat cells and this supply of estrogen is crucial to a woman's health as she ages. The uterus and the cervix also remain important because they continue to be stimulated during sexual intercourse, leading to a stronger orgasm in many women. To remove these organs without good cause not only puts women at risk from the surgical procedure itself, but may also damage the quality of their lives as they age.

Therefore, major surgery to remove your reproductive organs should not be performed for any of the following reasons:

1) as a sterilization technique—tubal ligation, involving blocking the Fallopian tubes to prevent conception, is safer and involves far fewer long-term side effects;

2) to prevent future, potential cancer in someone without a previous medical history of, or a strong hereditary tendency toward, such a condition;

3) to remove small, asymptomatic uterine fibroids (see below for more information about fibroids);

4) to treat mild unexplained or dysfunctional uterine bleeding, especially if other methods such as hormonal therapy with progesterone has not yet been attempted.

Before we discuss the conditions that may indeed warrant surgical removal of the female sex organs—and there are many— it is important to clarify our terms. Although some people assume that the term "total hysterectomy" refers to the removal of all sex organs, it is more complicated than that:

total hysterectomy refers to the removal of the uterus and cervix;

subtotal hysterectomy refers to the removal of the uterus only;

total hysterectomy and bilateral oophorectomy denotes the removal of the uterus, cervix, and both ovaries;

total hysterectomy and oophorectomy refers to the removal of the uterus, cervix, and one ovary (see Figure 4, below).

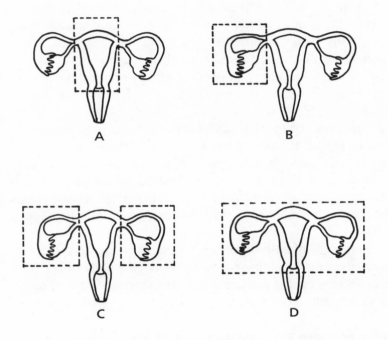

A   B

C   D

FIGURE 4 Partial and total hysterectomies. (A) Total hysterectomy: only the uterus and no other organs are removed. In salpingo-oophorectomy, one ovary and fallopian tube (B) or both ovaries and both tubes (C) are removed. (D) Total hysterectomy plus salpingo-oophorectomy.

In order to simplify our discussion here, the term *hysterectomy* will be used to describe the removal of the uterus and cervix only and *hysterectomy and bilateral oophorectomy* to describe the removal of the ovaries as well as the uterus and cervix.

OOPHORECTOMIES

Although hysterectomies and oophorectomies are serious operations that should not be undertaken lightly, there are several conditions that may indeed make it necessary to remove your reproductive organs. Generally speaking, your *ovaries* should be removed only under these circumstances:

Ovarian cancer

Ovarian cancer affects about one in seventy American women today and is more common in postmenopausal women. In its early stages, it produces few noticeable symptoms and is most often discovered during a routine pelvic exam. As the cancer progresses, pain and swelling usually occur; more than 75 percent of all ovarian cancers are diagnosed at this late stage of disease.

Treatment of ovarian cancer involves surgery to remove the ovaries and, if the cancer has spread, also the uterus, fallopian tubes, and nearby lymph glands. If the disease is caught in its earliest stages, the cancer may be limited to just one ovary. In that case, especially if the patient is still in her childbearing years, the surgeon may opt to remove just one ovary and its fallopian tube.

Surgery is often followed by radiation and/or chemotherapy to remove any remaining cancer cells from the body. When ovarian cancer is caught early, the five year survival rate is about 60 to 80 percent.

Some estrogen-dependent cancers of the uterus or breast

As discussed in Chapter Four, certain cancers of the breast and uterus are stimulated by the presence of estrogen. In order to treat such cancer, it may be necessary to remove the ovaries to remove the source of circulating estrogen. However, some estrogen-dependent breast cancers can now be treated with antihormonal therapy, which suppresses the action of estrogen on cancerous breast tissue.

As discussed in Chapter Four, the connection between breast cancer and estrogen is particularly problematic. About 60 percent of all women with breast cancer have tumors that contain greater than normal levels of estrogen and/or progesterone receptors on the surface of their breast tissue cells. Doctors test for the presence of estrogen/progesterone receptors when the biopsy is first performed on the mass or lump discovered in the breast.

In order to treat estrogen-dependent cancers, which may also occur in the endometrium, most physicians recommend a bilateral oophorectomy. However, a move away from oophorectomies for some estrogen-dependent cancers is now underway as antihormonal therapy is gaining favor among many in the medical community. Antihormonal therapy, primarily with a drug called tamoxifen (marketed in this country under the brand name Nolvadex), works to suppress estrogen stimulation of breast tissue and thereby halt the growth of tumors. This form of therapy is given to women once the malignant tumor has been surgically removed from the breast.

Tamoxifen works to prevent new tumors from forming by binding to the estrogen receptors on the cancerous or potentially cancerous cells; by doing so, tamoxifen prevents estrogen from stimulating the growth of these cells. In addition, once tamoxifen binds to the cancer cells, it works within the cells' nuclei to keep the cells from dividing. Eventually, the cancerous cells die altogether.

For most premenopausal women, the side effects of tamoxifen include minor menopausal symptoms, including hot flashes, fluid retention, and menstrual irregularities. However, in most cases, since the ovaries still produce estrogen, the bones, circulatory system, and vaginal tissues remain stimulated by regular hormonal activity. And, when treatment with tamoxifen ends—usually after five to ten years—periods return to normal and a woman is perfectly capable of conceiving, carrying, and delivering a baby.

In postmenopausal women, treatment with tamoxifen brings similar benefits to bones and blood vessels as those provided by estrogen replacement, at least in part because the drug appears to stimulate extra estrogen production in the body.

Although tamoxifen is not a miracle drug and is not effective for every woman or every type of breast cancer, it may be an option for you. If not, another drug, called Lupron or Megace, is also available. Megace works to suppress the luteinizing hormone (LH), which thus prevents the follicle from developing and estrogen from being produced; in effect this produces a chemical oopherectomy, since the ovaries no longer produce hormones. Once treatment with Megace stops, however, ovarian function eventually returns to normal.

Every day, new breakthroughs in cancer treatment and gynecology emerge. If your doctor suggests an oophorectomy to treat breast cancer, talk to him or her about these new approaches.

Severe ovarian cysts

Ovarian cysts, which are fluid-filled sacs, are fairly common and most require no treatment other than careful monitoring. In rare cases, ovarian cysts may become so large that they cause abnormal bleeding and pain. If these symptomatic cysts are small enough, a relatively minor procedure that drains the cysts with an instrument called a laparoscope (discussed in more detail later in this chapter in the section "Surgical Techniques") may alleviate the condition. In more serious cases, surgery is required to remove the cysts or, if the cysts are too large and invasive, to remove either one or both ovaries.

Severe endometriosis

Endometriosis affects about 10 to 15 percent of American women of childbearing age. It occurs when bits of the uterine lining (endometrium) escape the uterus and attach themselves to other pelvic organs. Most often, the implants form on the outside of the ovaries, fallopian tubes, or the uterus itself. When stimulated by the monthly cycle of estrogen production, the endometrial tissue—no matter where it is located—may begin to swell, pressing on the organs to which it is attached.

Most cases of endometriosis are so mild that they require no treatment, but for some women, it is a progressive disease that becomes more painful and debilitating over time. Many women find that taking birth control pills, which regulate hormonal production, relieves most symptoms. In other cases, physicians may decide to halt menstruation altogether through the use of certain hormones. Without estrogen stimulation, endometrial implants eventually wither and die, and often the condition never recurs. If drug treatment fails, surgery to remove the endometrial tissue—while leaving the affected organs—will be attempted. Only if these measures fail to alleviate the symptoms should the ovaries and/or uterus be removed.

HYSTERECTOMIES

As stated above, the removal of your uterus and cervix is one of the most common operations performed in the United States today, *and* it is estimated that nearly 50 percent of these surgeries are unnecessary. What conditions warrant the removal of your womb?

Endometrial cancer of the uterus

One of the most common cancers that afflict American women today, cancer of the uterine lining most often occurs in women between the ages of fifty and seventy. As discussed in Chapter Four, treatment with unopposed estrogen may increase the risk of endometrial cancer, but estrogen-progesterone therapy promotes no such increased risk.

Endometrial cancer is usually slow growing and apt to be localized when it is discovered. The five year survival rate for this type of cancer is more than 88 percent when discovered in its early stages; even if it has spread to adjacent tissues, the rate is 75 percent. In nearly all cases of endometrial cancer, removal of the uterus is recommended, as well as follow up treatment with radiation and/or chemotherapy.

Large uterine fibroids

About 20 percent of women over the age of thirty-five develop uterine fibroids. Also called leiomyomas, myomas, or fibromyomas, fibroids are benign tumors that develop within the uterine wall or attach themselves to it. Fibroids are usually stimulated to grow by the presence of estrogen. Therefore, women on birth control pills or estrogen replacement therapy are more prone to develop fast-growing fibroids than women who do not take hormones.

In most cases, fibroids cause no symptoms and eventually disappear without intervention. In other cases, they cause heavy and prolonged menstrual periods that can lead to anemia as well as pain or pressure in the lower abdomen or lower back.

Treatment of fibroids depends on the symptoms involved. In some cases, small fibroids can be removed during a D & C—dilation and curettage (see Appendix I for further details). In a procedure called a myomectomy, the surgeon removes the fibroids from the uterus, then repairs the tissue to preserve the womb; although complicated and a bit riskier than a hysterectomy, a successful myomectomy allows a woman to remain able to conceive and bring a child to term. Like ovarian cysts, fibroids may return again and again. If they cause severe symptoms, removal of the uterus may be indicated as a last resort.

Severe pelvic inflammatory disease

Pelvic inflammatory disease (PID), or infection of the fallopian tubes, ovaries, uterus, and cervix, affects about one million American women every year. Although most cases are caused by sexually transmitted bacteria, other cases can be traced to poorly sterilized surgical equipment used to perform D & C's or other gynecological procedures. PID causes severe pain and tenderness in the lower abdomen, pain during intercourse, heavier than usual periods, and, in advanced cases, vomiting and fever. If untreated, PID can cause abscesses to develop on the fallopian tubes and ovaries, eventually leading to sterility. Peritonitis, an inflammation of the membrane that lines the abdominal cavity, may also occur.

Treatment for PID involves medication with antibiotics and bed rest. If the symptoms are severe and chronic, hysterectomy may be the only way to alleviate them.

Uterine prolapse

As described in Chapter Four, the muscles that hold the pelvic organs may become distended and weak as we lose estrogen and as we age. When this occurs to an extreme degree, pelvic organs, including the uterus, may drop—or prolapse—into the vaginal wall.

Although minor prolapses are common and rarely require treatment, if the uterus extends far enough, surgery may be necessary. In most cases, your doctor will recommend a surgical procedure known as vaginal repair in which the surgeon elevates the prolapsed uterus into place and tightens the muscles of the pelvis. In rare cases of severely weakened and stretched muscles, a hysterectomy is advised.

Severe endometriosis that doesn't respond to other treatment
See above under "Oophorectomies."

Excessive uterine bleeding
There are several causes of abnormal uterine bleeding, including most of the conditions discussed above. In some cases, dysfunctional uterine bleeding may be the culprit. As a woman passes through menopause, her ovaries begin to produce estrogen and progesterone in a very erratic and unpredictable fashion. If progesterone is not produced as often or in high enough quantities, the lining of her uterus will grow to an abnormal size under constant estrogen stimulation. When it does slough off and fall away as it would during a normal period, she may experience prolonged and heavy bleeding. The most common treatment for this type of uterine bleeding involves dosages of progesterone to counteract the estrogen produced by the ovaries.

In some cases, the cause of excessive bleeding remains unknown. If uncontrolled, it can cause severe anemia and may prevent you from leading a normal life. If treatment with progesterone or with a uterine scraping, a D & C, does not alleviate the condition, your gynecologist may have no choice but to remove your uterus.

SURGICAL TECHNIQUES
Hysterectomies and other procedures to remove tumors, fibroids, and endometrial tissue are performed in a variety of ways. One of the most common procedures is the D & C, or dilation and curettage. A D & C involves first widening the cervical opening with dilators, then scraping and removing tissue

with an instrument known as a curette. Your doctor may perform a D & C as a diagnostic tool, since it allows him or her to check the uterine lining for growths with the curette. In addition, a D & C may be used as a surgical technique to remove small growths that may be causing pain or abnormal bleeding.

If major surgery is required to remove larger growths or to remove the uterus and/or ovaries, your doctor now has a number of different surgical techniques from which to choose. Most hysterectomies—about 75 percent—involve abdominal surgery: an incision is made in the lower abdomen either horizontally just above the pubic hair or vertically from the navel down. From this vantage point, tumors or organs are removed through the abdominal incision. In other cases, particularly those involving a hysterectomy to correct uterine prolapse, a vaginal procedure is performed in which organs are removed through an incision made at the top of the vagina. Both abdominal and vaginal surgeries require general anesthesia and a five to seven day hospital stay. Recuperation from abdominal surgery can be painful and time-consuming, involving about a month of bed rest at home for most women. Vaginal surgery results in less scarring, however, and tends to be easier to recover from than abdominal surgery.

A relatively new technique involving laser technology is gaining ground among gynecological surgeons. It involves an instrument called a laparoscope, a narrow tube with a light at one end and a series of lenses inside—rather like a tiny camera. About the size of magic marker, the laparoscope can be inserted in a tiny incision in the abodomen. To give the scope more room to explore, harmless gas is usually pumped into the abdomen. The camera on the tip of the laparoscope then sends a magnified image of the organs under inspection to the doctor, who peers in from the other end of the tube or watches as the image appears on a television monitor hooked up to the scope. Laparoscopes can be fitted with lenses that magnify an image fifteen times or more.

If the surgeon discovers any signs of trouble—fibroids or endometriosis, for example—another tiny incision is made and a laser is inserted. The laser beam, which is a highly concentrated light, is then aimed at the diseased tissue which is destroyed by the beam of light. In one laser procedure, called LAVH or laparoscopically assisted vaginal hysterectomy, the laser severs the uterus from connecting tissue, allowing the surgeon to remove it easily through the vagina. Laser-assisted laparoscopy is particularly useful in performing tubal ligations and in removing fibroids, ectopic pregnancies, and endometrial implants.

Surgeons find that laser surgery performed with the aid of the laparoscope involves not only less external scarring, but less internal scarring as well. For younger women who still want children, this technique may mean the difference between sterility and fertility following surgery. For all women, it means less time in the hospital and, frequently, a lower hospital bill. According to a September, 1992 article in *Glamour* magazine, the average cost of an abdominal hysterectomy is about $7,000; the same procedure performed with a laparoscope runs about $4,500.

Despite its many benefits, laparoscopy is not appropriate for all types of gynecological surgery. It is best performed on women known to have benign conditions, such as early-stage endometriosis and fibroids. To treat cervical, uterine, and ovarian cancer or to remove large masses of tissue, however, most doctors prefer to perform conventional abdominal surgery. If you are facing a hysterectomy for any reason, talk to your doctor about which method of surgery is the best one for you.

WHAT TO EXPECT

As discussed in Chapter One, only a bilateral oophorectomy results in certain, immediate menopause. When both your ovaries are removed, your supply of estrogen and progesterone is completely depleted. Within just a few days of surgery, you may experience hot flashes, night sweats, and other symptoms of menopause. You will no longer ovulate or have menstrual periods. In addition, the longer you are without estrogen, the higher risk you'll have of developing osteoporosis and cardiovascular disease. Unless you are being treated for an estrogen-dependent cancer, you will probably be prescribed HRT soon after surgery.

On the other hand, if only one of your ovaries is removed, you will continue to menstruate normally and be able to conceive and bear a child. Even in postmenopausal women, it is advised to limit the surgery to one ovary whenever possible. As discussed, the ovaries continue to play a role in the health of the body after menopause.

If you undergo a hysterectomy involving the removal of the uterus and cervix, you will probably continue to produce estrogen and progesterone in normal amounts. In rare cases, the surgical procedure may cut off the blood supply to the ovaries, causing them to stop functioning and menopausal symptoms to ensue. Usually such a condition is temporary; normal ovarian function resumes once the body is fully healed. If you are postmenopausal and taking HRT, your hysterectomy should not interfere with your therapy or vice versa.

WHAT TO ASK YOUR DOCTOR

If you have been diagnosed with one of the conditions listed above, and all other forms of treatment have failed to correct it, your doctor may decide that surgery to remove the affected organ or organs is necessary. Before you go ahead, you may want to consider getting a second opinion, preferably from a surgeon with whom your own doctor is unaffiliated. (And keep in mind—many insurance policies *require* a second opinion.) If possible, talk to an internist or gynecologist rather than a surgeon; surgeons, after all, are trained primarily in surgical techniques and their knowledge of other treatments may be limited. In addition, there are almost as many different medical approaches to gynecological problems as there are physicians. Your doctor should have no objection to your seeking another opinion; if he or she does object, you may want to consider finding another doctor who is more open to your needs.

The questions you'll want to ask both your own and the consulting physician include:

1) Are there any alternatives to surgery we have not yet tried? If so, what are the side effects and risks associated with them?
2) What will happen to me if I decide against the surgery? Will the condition lessen, disappear, or get worse?

3) What type of surgery is best for me (abdominal, vaginal, or laser)?

4) What are the risks and benefits of this type of surgery?

5) What are the potential complications or side effects of surgery?

6) How long will I expect to be recuperating? How much pain will I be in?

7) How will the outcome of surgery affect the rest of my life and my overall health?

If, after receiving answers to all these questions, you decide to go ahead with the surgery, you can rest assured that the decision you've made is an informed one. Despite the risks and the side effects, which may include premature menopause, you'll know that you are improving your health and quality of life by having a hysterectomy and/or oophorectomy.

LIVING WITH PREMATURE MENOPAUSE

Quite apart from the physical aspects of premature menopause and/or hysterectomies at any age, most women also feel a sense of emotional loss when their reproductive organs are no longer viable. Even women who have been post-menopausal for many years before having their ovaries or uterus removed report feelings of depression and sadness after surgery. Feel free to talk to your doctor about your feelings or, even better, to join a support group of women who have undergone a similar procedure or illness. You'd be surprised how much you have to share with one another.

No matter what has caused your ovaries to fail, you will no doubt suffer from one symptom or another related to the ensuing lack of female sex hormones. In the next chapter, you'll learn everything you need to know about coping with these symptoms whether or not you decide to replace those hormones with HRT.

CHAPTER 6

TAKING CHARGE: SELF-HELP STRATEGIES

"The change of life," a rather over-used euphemism for menopause, is in fact an apt description of what happens to a woman when she passes this milestone. In addition to any emotional upheavals that may take place concurrently, her physical life fundamentally changes when her ovaries no longer function to produce sex hormones. At the same time, five decades of wear and tear begin to show on virtually every part of a woman's body, from her hair and skin to her internal organs.

As outlined in Chapter Five, hormone replacement therapy has been shown to effectively forestall, allay, or reverse most of these changes. However, many women, for either medical or personal reasons, choose not to take HRT and it is largely for them that this chapter on dealing with the effects of menopause and aging has been written. Of course, every woman—on HRT or not—can benefit from knowing the fundamentals of good dental and eye care or learning how to make sex more enjoyable as she ages.

Because each woman experiences menopause in a different way, this chapter has been organized as a kind of an alphabetical smorgasbord of symptoms, side effects, and treatments. You may choose to read only those that affect you personally—if you suffer from hot flashes, for instance, you may want to skip ahead to learn tips on how best to cope with them—or you may decide to read through the whole chapter and then go back to pore over those with the most significance to you at this time.

As you are no doubt aware, proper nutrition and regular exercise are the mainstays of human health at any age. Because of their importance, we've devoted a separate chapter to discuss each of them at length. For example, although you'll learn that calcium may help prevent osteoporosis here, Chapter Seven will teach you which foods contain the most calcium and give you tips on how to add those foods to your daily diet.

Again, every woman passes through menopause in a unique way and some may require more medical intervention than others. The suggestions below will help you to make your own change of life as easy and as pleasant as possible, but it's important that you speak directly and openly with your physician about your own experience and personal needs.

YOUR A TO Z GUIDE TO MENOPAUSE
Symptoms, Side Effects, and Treatment

Below are some of the topics covered in this chapter.

Arthritis

Atherosclerosis

Breast changes

    sagging tissue

    changes in size

    cosmetic surgery

Dental care

Depression

Hair care

    body hair, increase of

    dry hair

    gray hair

    thinning hair

Hot flashes

Sex

    contraception

    libido, loss of

    muscle tone, loss of

    painful

Skin changes

    age spots

    dry skin

    wrinkles

    cosmetic surgery

Sleep disturbances

Smoking

Urinary incontinence

Urinary tract and

    vaginal infections

ARTHRITIS

Arthritis, or inflammation of the joints, is one of the most common disorders in the United States, affecting more than thirty-six million people. Although arthritis is caused by a variety of influences and can strike at any age, one form of it affects older people more than any other segment of the population.

Osteoarthritis is the gradual degeneration of cartilage, the tissue that surrounds the joints to form a protective cushion around the bones. As cartilage degenerates, aches, pains, and swelling result. Eventually, the cartilage may wear away completely, exposing bone to serious injury. The result of the repetitive use of joints over time, osteoarthritis eventually affects almost everyone over the age of sixty to some degree. The joints most commonly affected include the vertebrae, knees, hip, neck, and fingers.

Because women tend to experience the first symptoms of osteoarthritis at about the same time that they pass through menopause, they often assume that their aches and pains are somehow connected to the loss of sex hormones. In fact, there may be some connection, since estrogen affects the production of steroids, substances that work to protect the joints from injury. However, since men and women suffer from the disease in about equal numbers at every age, menopause plays a relatively minor role in most cases.

Estrogen does play a major role in the development of rheumatoid arthritis, a particularly disabling form of arthritis that occurs in three times as many women as men. In March 1986, the *Journal of the American Medical Association* reported on a study conducted at Erasmus University in the Netherlands that showed that women who took estrogen replacement had nearly a 25 percent less chance of developing rheumatoid arthritis than women who did not. If rheumatoid arthritis runs in your family, or if you already suffer from this disease, talk to your doctor about estrogen.

Treatment for most cases of osteoarthritis involves taking anti-inflammatory drugs such as aspirin or ibuprofen and keeping the joints strong and flexible with stretching and range-of-motion exercises. If osteoarthritis affects your spine or your knees, however, weight-bearing exercises such as jogging or tennis should be avoided. You may want to visit a physical therapist familiar with osteoarthritis to devise an exercise plan that's right for you.

In rare cases of advanced disease, surgery to replace a damaged hip or knee joint or to remove particles of bone damaging cartilage may be performed. For more information about osteo- or other types of arthritis, contact your local chapter of the Arthritis Foundation. (See Appendix II: Resources.)

ATHEROSCLEROSIS

As discussed at length in Chapter Three, atherosclerosis is one of the most insidious and damaging diseases affecting older Americans today. Although it is likely that some degree of vessel damage is bound to occur as we age, there is no doubt that a proper diet—one low in saturated fat and high in complex carbohydrates—and regular exercise will help prevent cardiovascular disease from ending or limiting our lives prematurely. Women who do not take HRT are at special risk of cardiovascular disease and should pay special attention to the information presented in Chapters Seven and Eight.

BREAST CHANGES

Like all other parts of her body, a woman's breasts change as she ages and, unfortunately, not often for the better. As discussed in Chapters Four and Five, the risk of developing breast cancer rises as you age. In fact, a recent report by the National Cancer Institute confirms the fact that more than 80 percent of all breast cancers occur in women over the age of fifty and that about 30 percent are fatal. Needless to say, regular self-exams and mammograms are a must for all women. (See Appendix I for more details.)

In addition to this serious health risk are cosmetic changes in the breasts that also come with age. Perhaps the most common body image complaint among older women is that their breasts begin to sag and lose their shape, while the skin covering the breasts becomes dry and wrinkly. Although some of these changes are related to the loss of estrogen stimulation and may be alleviated with HRT, most women need to pay special attention to their breasts in order to keep them firm and supple.

Sagging breasts, for instance, result from the fact that muscles and ligaments meant to support breast tissue begin to lose elasticity and strength as we get older. The large muscles of the chest, called the pectoralis major, and the upper back muscles, called the trapezius, are the main structures involved in supporting the breasts. The only way to prevent loss of tone in these muscles is to exercise them: standard or modified push-ups and chest-arm isometrics are among the best exercises for the pectorals and trapezius muscles. Free weights and/or Nautilus or other weight-training machines designed to work these muscles will also help to maintain or create breast support. (See Chapter Eight for more details.)

The size and shape of breasts change because fat cells tend to diminish and milk glands to shrink with lack of estrogen and hormonal stimulation, making the breasts smaller and less supple. Other women find that their breasts become larger and more pendulous as they age. Unfortunately, apart from taking HRT, there is really not much you can do to prevent such changes from taking place. Wearing support bras, however, will help you feel more comfortable, especially while you exercise.

Some women unhappy or uncomfortable with their breasts decide that plastic surgery is a healthy and positive option for them. Those with particularly large and/or pendulous breasts may opt to have their breasts reduced. In this type of surgery, cuts are made into the fold under the breasts, excess fat and skin is removed, and the skin is sutured back into place. The breasts then look and feel firmer.

Women whose breasts have become smaller, due to surgery for breast cancer or through hormonal and age related changes, may opt for breast reconstruction or augmentation. All plastic surgery procedures are complicated and involve many risks as well as benefits that go far beyond the scope of this book. Discuss the matter with your physician and check the "Plastic Surgery" section listed in Appendix II for more information.

DENTAL CARE

About 50 percent of all Americans have lost several of their adult teeth by the time they reach the age of seventy. The number one cause of tooth loss in older Americans is periodontal disease—disease that affects the structures that surround the teeth, including the gums, ligaments, and bone—caused by a buildup of plaque. Plaque, a sticky, bacteria-filled film, forms on your teeth every day. If not removed on a regular basis, bacterial plaque may infect the gums, causing a disease known as gingivitis, or inflammation of the gums. Over time, plaque may harden into a substance called tartar, which may further inflame and infect gum tissue until tooth sockets become so weak and enlarged that teeth loosen and fall out.

As discussed in Chapter Three, another common cause of tooth loss after menopause is osteoporosis of the jaw bone. According to the National Osteoporosis Foundation, women in their sixties with osteoporosis were three times as likely to have dentures as women without the disease. Maintaining a diet rich in calcium and/or taking calcium supplements may help prevent some bone loss, but it appears that estrogen replacement remains the best option for women at risk for osteoporosis.

Controlling plaque buildup is more difficult after menopause because we tend to produce less saliva, which has a natural cleansing effect on the teeth. That means that brushing and flossing after every meal—or at least twice a day—is essential. Many dentists also recommend gum massage by an irrigating instrument, such as a Waterpik. In addition, you might want to try one of the toothpastes or mouth washes designed to prevent plaque buildup recently approved by the American Dental Association and the Food and Drug Administration. Dental exams and cleaning should occur at least once a year; if you have a tendency to build plaque, try to visit your dentist every six months for a cleaning.

If you do lose one or more teeth due to periodontal disease, you have more options than ever when it comes to replacing them. If the root of your tooth remains firmly attached to your jawbone (and your jawbone is unaffected by osteoporosis), your dentist will file down the remaining enamel and hollow out the infected pulp from the canal that leads to the root. Once the canal is thoroughly cleaned, it is filled permanently with sterilized material and covered with a crown, a synthetic material designed to match the surrounding teeth. This process is commonly known as a root canal and crown replacement.

If more than one tooth in a row is involved, your dentist may create either a fixed bridge (a process resembling the one described above over more than one tooth) or a removable bridge. A removable bridge consists of synthetic teeth attached to a metal framework designed to snap into place using clasps around the remaining teeth. In this case, the roots of your teeth are removed as well as the enamel and infected pulp. Removable bridges tend to be less expensive than fixed bridges but are usually not as comfortable or durable. If tooth loss becomes widespread, you may eventually require full dentures.

Some people are able to avoid removable bridges and dentures through a new technique called dental implantation. This procedure involves implanting artificial teeth directly into the jawbone. Although dental implantation is currently rather expensive, it is an option worth discussing with your dentist should you face the loss of your teeth. Losing one's teeth is often an emotionally devastating as well as physically painful event and we all should do whatever we can to prevent this from occurring.

DEPRESSION

Women get hit with a double whammy when it comes to depression. First of all, throughout our lives, we have a greater tendency toward the condition than do men, largely because our hormones exert enormous influence over our moods. Second, just at the time when upsetting events occur more often—the death of a loved one, divorce, loss of self-esteem due to body image changes—in both men and women, women experience even more profound hormonal changes than ever before as they lose ovarian function.

Does this mean that women are doomed to suffer depression once they pass menopause? In fact, that appears not to be the case. According to a study done in Baltimore in the early 1980s by the Eastern Baltimore Mental Health Unit, people between the ages of eighteen and sixty-four had three times the incidence of major depressions than those in the sixty-five to seventy-four age group. Nevertheless, depression is more widespread than we may tend to think among older Americans: according to the National Institutes of Mental Health, approximately 10 to 15 percent of people over the age of fifty-five suffer at least one bout of depression; many more cases may be misdiagnosed or overlooked.

The most commonly asked question about depression involves defining the condition more precisely: when does feeling sad turn into depression? Indeed, experiencing occasional, brief periods of despondency, grief, and/or self-doubt is common, quite normal, and, in many ways demonstrates a healthy response to life's challenges. However, when these feelings persist and cause radical changes in your day-to-day life, you may require medical intervention to help you cope. (Table 2 below will help you to recognize the difference between normal sadness and depression.)

TABLE 2

Differences Between Depression and Normal Sadness

Features	Normal Sadness	Depression
Recent difficult or tragic life event	Common	Unusual
Family history of depression	Absent	Present
Mood variation	Depression worse late in the day	Depression worse in the morning
Sleep disturbances	Difficulty in falling asleep but remains asleep	Middle of the night or early morning insomnia
Appetite	May be increased or decreased; mild or no weight loss	Little interest in food; rapid weight loss
Physical ailments	Fewer and less severe	Many and more severe
Physical and mental activity	Mild slowing or, more rarely, agitation	Moderate to severe slowing
Attitude	Self-pity, pessimism, but no loss of self-esteem	Self-blame, remorse, guilt, complete loss of self-esteem
Interest	Mild-to-moderate loss, but usually able to work	Pervasive loss of interest or pleasure in everything
Suicidal behavior or thoughts	Relatively uncommon	Common

Source: Reprinted from *Health and Nutrition Newsletter*, (Columbia University School of Public Health) Vol. 2, no. 10.

If you suffer from true depression, your doctor will most likely prescribe an antidepressant, such as Elavil or Prozac, that is designed to influence brain chemistry in order to lighten your dark moods. These drugs can be addictive, however, and should be taken only under the continued care of your physician. Drugs alone are not usually enough to dispel depression; psychotherapy may be required to help you discover the root causes of your depression and find appropriate solutions. In severe cases, electroconvulsive therapy (shock therapy), which involves stimulating brain chemicals with a mild electric current, may be indicated.

Even if your blue moods are not serious enough to require medical intervention, they can be annoying, frustrating, and, yes, depressing! These feelings can stem from any number of sources as you pass through menopause: many marriages fail at this time, children leave home, careers come to an end, and the physical effects of aging begin to show on your face and body. Both women and men must now face up to goals that may never be realized, dreams still out of reach, challenges that have yet to be met. As down to earth as these realizations may be, they often come as a disappointing shock from which it is difficult to recover.

How do you fight the blues? First of all, review your diet and exercise patterns. If you're not eating enough, you could be feeling lethargic simply because you're not properly nourished. An excess of caffeine or sugar could be responsible for at least some of your irritability and insomnia. Exercise may get your motor running up to speed as well. In addition to keeping your heart healthy and your brain nourished, it also stimulates the production and release of endorphins, chemicals produced by the central nervous system that suppress pain while inducing feelings of euphoria.

Without a doubt, your best protection from the blues is to stay active and involved, even if what you'd rather do is curl up into the fetal position and watch old movies for the rest of your life. Find a new hobby, bury yourself in an exciting project at work or at home, join a health club, or go on an exotic vacation. Learn to cook Chinese food or take a writing class. As trivial as these activities may seem when you're feeling low, simply getting out and breathing fresh air—both physically and intellectually—is the very best prescription for you to follow.

If your feelings of sadness, loss, and low self-esteem persist, it's essential that you treat your symptoms seriously. Many women suffer from mild to moderate depression without seeking help for fear that they'll appear neurotic or "crazy." If you haven't been able to get yourself up and out of the doldrums, take the time to answer these questions. Have you been experiencing any of the following symptoms for more than a day or two at a time:

____ Insomnia or excessive sleepiness?

____ Loss of appetite and weight loss?

____ Low energy level?

____ Loss of self-esteem?

____ Decreased productivity?

____ Decreased attention span or increased confusion?

____ Withdrawal from social interaction?

____ Loss of enjoyment, even in activities that once brought you pleasure?

____ Frequent bouts of irritability or anger?

____ Self-reproach or inappropriate guilt?

____ Recurrent thought of suicide and death?

____ Sense of helplessness and gloom?

If you have answered in the affirmative to three or more of these questions, you may be suffering from depression. If so, you should seek help from your physician immediately. Unlike normal feelings of sadness and grief, depression is a serious condition frequently requiring medical intervention.

HAIR CARE

Hardly immune from either hormonal disturbances or the ravages of time, the hair on your body and on your head changes as you pass through menopause; to keep it healthy and attractive may well require some extra effort on your part. If you're like most women, however, you'll find that the benefits you reap in terms of heightened self-esteem are well worth whatever special attention you must now pay.

Body hair

One of the most annoying changes that take place after menopause is the increase in darker, thicker body hair that results from the imbalance between female and male hormones created by the loss of estrogen. Many women notice that the hair on their upper lips and chins, around the nipples, and on their forearms and thighs are particularly susceptible to this often disturbing new trend.

Luckily, there are many simple solutions to this problem. If you decide to take HRT, you'll find that body hair growth returns to normal within just a few weeks. If HRT is not right for you, several solutions are available. Commercial bleaches can be applied that camouflage dark hairs by lightening them to a shade of white or blond. If you choose this method, read the package directions carefully, and be sure to perform a 24-hour patch test to determine if the product is safe for you to use.

Shaving is the easiest and least expensive method to remove hair from your legs, underarms, bikini areas, and even your upper lip. To be effective, it must be done often—at least every few days (every day on your face)—and with a very sharp razor and shaving cream to prevent nicks and cuts.

Many women prefer to remove hair from these areas with depilatories, chemical creams that dissolve the hair and break it off beneath the skin. The effects of depilatories last longer (about a week) than those derived from shaving and also tend to make the skin feel softer and smoother. However, some women find that the chemicals involved irritate the skin, causing rashes and/or a stinging sensation.

To remove hair around the nipples and eyebrows, most women decide that tweezing is the most effective method. Because it involves literally pulling each hair out by the root one by one, however, tweezing can be quite painful and tedious. For larger areas with extensive hair growth, such as the legs and bikini areas, waxing is another option. Waxing involves applying a liquid wax to the skin, allowing it to set, then pulling it off in one quick motion. Along with the wax comes body hair, which is pulled out by its roots. Waxes, like depilatories, may be irritating to the skin or cause burns if not properly applied. Although home waxing kits are available, the procedure is best performed in a salon.

The only permanent solution to the overgrowth of body hair is electrolysis, which involves destroying the hair root by inserting a fine needle into the hair follicle and zapping the root with a weak electrical current. Like tweezing, electrolysis is tedious and painful and is usually only effective on small areas such as the chin, upper lip, or eyebrows. Moreover, it is usually expensive and can be dangerous if not performed by a trained professional.

Head hair

A head of shiny, soft hair is a hallmark not only of an attractive woman but a healthy woman as well. Although certain changes are bound to occur due to the loss of estrogen and the aging process, it is possible to keep your hair looking lustrous if you eat properly, exercise regularly, and pay special attention to your changing needs.

Hair, like skin tissue, has a tendency to become drier with the loss of estrogen. If you decide against using HRT, you can make up for some of this loss of moisture by making sure you drink plenty of water (at least eight glasses a day), avoid overexposure to the sun, and eat a balanced diet (see Chapter Seven) that includes an appropriate amount of protein and vitamins A, B, C, D, and E, which may have especially good effects on your hair. External preparations, including commercial hair moisturizers and homemade preparations that use vegetable oils, avocados, or other oil-rich products, may also help keep the hair supple and shiny.

For both men and women, the cardinal sign of aging is gray hair. Hair turns gray because we produce less and less pigment—the substance that gives our hair color—the older we get. Although a tendency toward early graying is hereditary, everyone eventually turns gray: by the age of fifty, more than half the population has gray hair and the percentage continues to grow with each decade of life.

If gray hair, which tends to be coarser and dryer than pigmented hair, is kept moist and shiny, it can be as attractive as any other color. In fact, with the right cut, gray hair can be dramatic and highly stylish. If you like your gray hair, you should feel under no obligation to change it to suit some arbitrary social standard that equates salt-and-pepper with old age. On the other hand, coloring one's hair with commercial dyes is safe and easy. In fact, many new preparations actually work to make your hair appear and feel thicker and more supple. Talk to your hairdresser about coloring your hair if you feel at all uncomfortable with the appearance of gray.

Although thinning hair tends to occur more often in men, many women past the age of menopause find that their hair has begun to thin out as well. As you may remember, the lack of estrogen-stimulation of the collagen surrounding the hair follicle only encourages the loss of hair; the fact that we tend to replenish lost hair less often the older we get only exacerbates the problem. To prevent excess hair loss, you should avoid using harsh chemicals that will weaken the hair shaft, limit the use of hair dryers and electric rollers that will dry out the hair and cause excess breakage, and use a proper hairbrush equipped with soft, rounded—not stiff or blunt—bristles.

HOT FLASHES

The number one symptom of menopause, experienced by at least 75 percent of all women, is the hot flash. As discussed in Chapter Two, hot flashes are caused by the effect of the hormonal imbalance on the hypothalamus. Although each woman experiences hot flashes in her own unique way, these episodes usually consist of excessive sweating, reddening of the skin, and an increase in body temperature. Hot flashes are annoying, frequently embarrassing, and often completely unpredictable. Luckily, about 65 percent of women with hot flashes find that they subside on their own after about a year or two. About 30 percent experience hot flashes for about five years and only a very small percentage have them for longer periods.

The quickest and most effective treatment for hot flashes is estrogen-progesterone replacement. If you decide that HRT is not right for you, however, there are several techniques that will help you minimize the occurrence of hot flashes and keep you as comfortable as possible when they do occur.

1) Keep track of how often and under what circumstances your hot flashes occur. That way, you'll be able to identify your hot flash "triggers": those foods, environmental conditions, and/or emotional situations that stimulate a hot flash reaction.

2) Stay cool and try to avoid dramatic swings in temperature. Many women find that they experience more frequent and severe hot flashes in the summer than in the winter. If you do not have an air-conditioned home or office, be sure to have a portable fan near you at all times when the temperature begins to climb. Dress in cool cottons and drink plenty of cool water.

Air-conditioning can prove to be a double-edged sword, however, as some women find that it is not heat per se that aggravates their hot flashes but any dramatic temperature change. Going from blistering heat into an air-conditioned building or room (or going from a toasty warm house into the bitter cold) can provoke the onset of a hot flash as well. If temperature swings bother you, try to mitigate them whenever possible by waiting a few minutes in a semicool lobby before entering an air-conditioned or heated store, office, or home.

3) Wear several layers of clothing, especially on the upper body. With an undershirt, blouse, and light sweater or jacket, for instance, you can remove or replace clothing as your temperature—or the temperature of your environment—increases and decreases. If you sweat excessively during a hot flash, you may want to carry an extra undershirt or blouse so you can change should your clothing become damp.

4) Choose to wear clothing made from cotton or other natural fibers, which tend to release heat and moisture rather than trap it between the fabric and the skin. New activewear fibers such as polypropylene may also help keep excess perspiration away from your skin.

5) Wear lighter makeup and moisturizers to avoid streaking and feeling sticky if you should perspire heavily during hot flashes. And the simpler the makeup the better: complicated eye makeup that includes several shadows, eyeliner, and mascara is difficult to both remove quickly or repair once it becomes smudged. Try cake eyeliner, which tends to be less water-soluble than liquid or pencil, and a waterproof mascara. Avoid heavy

powders, sticky lip gloss, and other products and stick to a light foundation, blush, and smooth lipstick.

6) Avoid spicy foods if you find that they trigger hot flashes. If you've ever perspired while eating foods flavored with pepper, cumin, or other hot spices, you know that what you eat can actually trigger your body to try to cool itself down. Because your hormones are already in flux, such an action can cause an especially severe hot flash. Check your log to see if a meal of Indian, Mexican, or other spicy cuisine preceded a hot flash. If so, avoid such food in the future.

7) Drink plenty of water, but avoid beverages that contain caffeine, sugar, and alcohol since these substances are hot flash triggers for many women. Instead, try herbal teas, especially those that are thought to have a relaxing effect on the body such as chamomile and ginseng. Since staying cool is often a priority for women suffering from hot flashes, try keeping a thermos of iced herbal tea nearby at all times.

8) Splash cool water on your face or plunge your hands into a basin of cool water to end a hot flash more quickly. Your body will sense that it has cooled down and may cease stimulating blood vessels to constrict and sweat glands to perspire in order to lower body temperature.

9) Avoid stressful situations. When your body perceives that it is in any kind of danger—from a missed deadline at work, for instance, or from something quite physical and imminent like an oncoming car—hormonal activity increases dramatically. Specifically, your adrenal medulla—an endocrine gland—releases the "fight or flight" stress hormones, norepinephrine and epinephrine, as well as cortisol and testosterone, when danger or stress is sensed by the brain. The job of epinephrine and norepinephrine is to stimulate heart and blood vessel action, in effect preparing the body for a physical fight against the perceived stress. Because your body's hormonal system is out of whack due to the loss of estrogen and progesterone, such a reaction could easily result in a hot flash.

Of course, avoiding stress is no easy task for most people, especially since a clear definition of stress does not exist. A woman who derives pleasure from a hectic day at the office, for instance, may find a day spent at the beach with nothing to do far more stressful than anything that might occur during her normal work day. As silly as it may seem, *trying* to relax can be a stressful activity in itself. If you relate relaxation with laziness, for instance, it's unlikely that you'll be able derive a sense of ease from taking a nap every afternoon. Nevertheless, it is important to find ways to relax, especially if you find that stress triggers your hot flashes.

During the past decade, considerable interest has been directed toward the question of whether the effects of stress on the body could be modified through behavior therapy. Biofeedback is one method that has received a good deal of attention. It was developed when studies showed that animals could control their autonomic functions, like blood pressure and heart rate, by being given a reward or a punishment. Physicians adapted those findings to design ways for humans to control unconscious functions through conscious thought.

There are many biofeedback methods. One involves monitoring patients with a machine equipped with lights similar to traffic lights. When blood pressure or body temperature increases, a special monitor will activate the lights on the machine to let the patient monitor her body's activities. The patient will learn to control her blood pressure, for instance, by consciously calming down if the pressure is too high or by thinking about stressful situations if the pressure is too low. The goal is for the patient to continue this method of control without the monitoring machine. Although no studies have been done that specifically test the effectiveness of biofeedback on hot flashes, there is every reason to believe that for women whose hot flashes are triggered by stress learning to relax will help to alleviate their condition.

Not all solutions to the problem of recognizing and relieving stress are so high-tech. For some, daily exercise will eliminate stress, while for others meditation is the answer. The relaxation response, developed by Boston physician Herbert Benson in the 1970s, relies on the tradition of transcendental meditation to evoke a calm, relaxed attitude in patients who are under stress. (For more information about biofeedback and meditation, see Appendix II: Resources.)

10) Exercise. A recent study of Swedish women who suffer from hot flashes reveals that regular, strenuous, aerobic exercise performed at least three times a week significantly diminishes the occurrence and severity of hot flash episodes. The exact mechanism by which exercise affects hot flashes is unknown, but scientists believe that the effect that aerobic activity has on blood pressure may be the link.

11) Keep smiling. Many women feel humiliated and embarrassed when they experience a hot flash in front of friends or strangers. Needless to say, this reaction only increases stress and makes it more likely that you'll perspire more, turn an even darker shade of red, and feel even more uncomfortable than if you attempted to pass the episode off with a smile. Remember, as annoying as they are, hot flashes are a natural, physiological reaction. Don't let them get you down.

SEXUAL CHANGES

Sexuality is an extremely personal and individual matter and every woman experiences sex in her own unique way. Although the media—especially television and movies—would have you think that sex is a woman's primary interest every day of her life, you must heed your own inner voice and instincts when it comes to your sexual behavior. If you enjoy sex and have an available partner, you should not fear that menopause will mean the end of your sex life. On the other hand, if sex simply does not interest you very much or if you do not have a sexual partner, you should not feel pressured to perform in a way that makes you feel uncomfortable.

The bottom line is: contrary to popular myth, the end of fertility does not signal the beginning of frigidity. The ability to have sex—and, more importantly, to *enjoy* sex—lasts for a lifetime.

It is true, however, that a variety of physical and emotional changes occur at menopause that may very well influence the way you experience sexual activity. As you may remember from Chapter Two, estrogen and progesterone profoundly affect a woman's sexual organs and the way they respond to sexual stimulation. As the rate at which you produce estrogen slowly diminishes over time, so too does the hormone's effect on the vagina, clitoris, and other organs involved in the sexual response.

After several months or years without estrogen, you may find sexual intercourse has become uncomfortable, even painful, because your vagina is dry and your vaginal wall is thin and lacks muscle tone and strength. In addition, you may find that everything takes a bit longer than it used to: as a young woman your vagina and labia (external genitalia) became lubricated in about fifteen to thirty seconds after being stimulated. After menopause, it may take up to five or ten minutes of foreplay before you become lubricated enough for comfortable penetration.

Unless you are aware that these changes are normal and are caused by a simple lack of estrogen, you and your partner may become frustrated and disappointed in the sexual experience. Your partner may think you are not aroused by him or that you are uninterested in sex; you may find the experience so uncomfortable that you turn away from sex altogether. Indeed, it appears that it is not the loss of estrogen per se that reduces a woman's libido as she ages, but rather the physical discomfort the loss of estrogen has on her sexual organs.

In addition, there are a number of psychosocial issues that may interfere with your ability to enjoy the sexual experience after you pass through menopause. A crucial barrier to a healthy sex life for many older women is the lack of an available partner. Death and divorce take their toll on the older woman, who then finds herself alone after several decades of marriage. In this day of sexually transmitted diseases, finding a new partner can seem especially difficult and frightening even to the most self-confident of women.

Which brings us to the self-confidence part of the equation. Feeling attractive and sexy is vital to a healthy, enjoyable sex life. But in these youth-obsessed times, many women over the age of fifty feel left out and over-the-hill. Perhaps as more and more television and movie executives—aging baby boomers that they are—hit the big "five-oh" themselves, we may see in our sitcoms, movies, and throughout our everyday lives a bit of respect for the sensuality and maturity that comes with age.

It should be noted that many women pass through menopause without feeling any different—physically or emotionally—about sex. However, if you are noticing any changes in your sex life at this time, try following some of these suggestions to raise your level of enjoyment:

1) Protect yourself from pregnancy and from sexually transmitted diseases. First of all, keep in mind that until you have ceased menstruating for at least one year and have received a confirmed diagnosis of menopause from your physician, you may still be fertile. As unlikely as it may seem, you can conceive a child at any age if you're still ovulating and having intercourse.

Talk to your gynecologist about what method of birth control is best for you at this time in your life. If you have been married for many years and both you and your spouse are monogamous, your risk of contracting a sexually transmitted disease (STD) is probably quite minimal. Therefore, any method of birth control, including the pill (if you don't smoke or have severe high blood pressure), diaphragm, IUD, or cervical cap will work for you. However, if you become intimate with a new partner or partners, it is important to protect yourself from the myriad STDs now circulating, including AIDS, gonorrhea, syphilis, and chlamydia, among others. Use a condom with a spermicidal jelly or cream each and every time you have sex—whether you need to protect yourself against pregnancy or not.

2) Enjoy intimacy. As stated above, it may take you longer to achieve arousal and orgasm today than it did when you were younger. Take advantage of this time by enjoying the sensual and romantic aspects of foreplay—and don't be afraid to ask for what you need. If your vagina and clitoris feel tender and sore, ask your partner to be more gentle during foreplay and intercourse.

At the same time, it is important for you to be sensitive to your partner's needs and potential difficulties. According to the Kinsey report released in the mid-1970s, about 25 percent of men experience a period of prolonged impotence during their sixties. Impotence can be caused by a variety of factors, including illnesses, such as diabetes and vascular disease, and drugs, such as those used to treat hypertension and depression. Keep in mind that if your partner is over the age of fifty, he too may need more time to become aroused and to ejaculate.

3) Lubricate liberally. If you decide against taking HRT, you may find that your vagina and vaginal wall need extra lubrication to make intercourse comfortable and exciting. If so, water-soluble lubricants, such as K-Y jelly, should help keep the area moist in all but the most severe cases of vaginal atrophy. Vegetable oil, coconut oil, and saliva are also good options. However, avoid any products made with petroleum, such as Vaseline, as they may be irritating to vaginal tissue.

4) Practice Kegel exercises. Developed more than forty years ago by Dr. A. M. Kegel, this system of exercises will help you strengthen the muscles—called the pubococcygeals—that support your pelvic organs and the vaginal tissues. Used primarily to help women with bladder control problems (see "Urinary incontinence" below), Kegel exercises also help to maintain the strength and responsiveness of the vaginal wall, thereby making intercourse more pleasurable for both women and their partners.

To locate the proper muscles involved, try this simple exercise: the next time you urinate, practice starting and stopping the flow of urine. The muscles you are contracting to stop the flow are the muscles you'll want to work during your Kegel exercise routine. You can perform Kegels lying down, standing up, or sitting. Simply tighten the pubococcygeal muscles for six to ten seconds, relax them for three seconds, then repeat the exercise as many times as you feel comfortable—up to about ten or twenty each set. The more sets of exercises you can do in a day, the stronger your muscles will become.

5) Stay sexually active. "Use it or lose it" appears to be an apt adage when it comes to sex and the older woman. A 1991 study, conducted by the Department of Obstetrics at the Robert Wood Johnson Medical School in New Brunswick, New Jersey, confirmed decades of research showing a direct correlation between continued sexual activity and both *desire for* and *enjoyment of* sexual activity.

In the New Jersey study, fifty-nine healthy, postmenopausal women between the ages of sixty and seventy were questioned about their sexual activity. Among the group, 66 percent were sexually active and 34 percent were abstinent. By far, those who were active reported having higher levels of sexual desire than their abstinent peers. Moreover, a pelvic examination revealed that the sexually active women showed fewer signs of vaginal atrophy than those women who remained abstinent. (It is interesting to note that the women who were active reported having had sex more often and enjoying sex to a greater degree when they were premenopausal than did the women who were abstinent after menopause.)

If you do not have a partner but still have sexual urges, you may want to consider masturbating. Although many of us were brought up to believe that self-stimulation was wrong or evil, masturbation is a perfectly natural activity, one that can bring us pleasure as well as keep both our sexual organs and our sense of sensuality healthy and vital. Many books, including *Our Bodies, Ourselves* and *The Joy of Sex*, are available to help you learn how to sexually explore your body, even if you've never done so in the past.

SKIN CHANGES

In 1990 alone, more than 49,000 face lifts, 79,000 eye-lifts, and 81,000 collagen injections were performed on the faces of mostly female Americans by doctors belonging to the American Society of Plastic and Reconstructive Surgeons. Those numbers confirm the fact that—rightly or wrongly—supple, young-looking skin is a top priority among Americans today.

Most every woman and man will first notice the signs of aging on the skin: the body's largest and most public organ. Because a woman's skin derives so much of its fullness and moisture from estrogen-dependent collagen, she will experience these changes much more quickly and severely than a man of the same age once her supply of estrogen is gone.

If you are able to take HRT, you'll probably find that your skin will remain healthier looking for a longer period of time than if you decide against therapy. However, with or without estrogen, keeping your skin healthy as you age requires maintaining good eating and exercise habits, protecting your skin from the sun and other pollutants, and learning to clean and moisturize your skin properly.

Avoid the sun and use sunscreen

According to estimates from some dermatologists, as much as 70 percent of the skin damage we associate with aging actually is caused by overexposure to the sun instead. Ultraviolet (UV) rays from the sun destroy the elastic fibers that provide support to the skin; without this support the skin sags and wrinkles. The sun also sucks moisture from the skin, leaving it feeling and looking dry and leathery. In addition, overexposure to the sun contributes to the development of skin cancer, especially in people with fair skin and a tendency to burn.

Fortunately, protection is available in the form of sunscreen preparations, which block most of the sun's UV rays. Whenever you are out in the sun, cover all exposed body parts with a sunscreen preparation with SPF (Sun Protection Factor) of 15 or higher. The SPF number represents the length of time you can stay in the sun before you burn, compared to the time it would take without sunscreen. By wearing a sunscreen with SPF 15, for instance, you can stay out in the sun fifteen times longer without getting a burn than you can with no protection. (If you're fair skinned and will be outdoors for long periods, choose an even higher SPF.) Apply the sunscreen at least thirty minutes before exposure to the sun, as it must penetrate the skin to be effective, and reapply it frequently and generously. If you plan to swim, make sure you use a waterproof sunscreen preparation. Be aware, however, that no matter how high their SPF, most sunscreens do not provide complete protection against all types of UV rays. Therefore, try to stay out of the sun during the middle of the day when the sun is at its strongest.

Stop smoking

In addition to its many other health hazards, cigarette smoking damages the skin in several different ways. First, nicotine is known to lower a woman's estrogen levels, thereby speeding up the aging process. Second, cigarette smoke is an external pollutant that clogs your pores with soot and chemicals. Finally, by causing blood vessels to contract, nicotine restricts the flow of blood and nutrients to the surface of the skin, leaving it undernourished and looking sallow and pale.

Drink plenty of water

All body cells need moisture to stay smooth and flexible; when skin cells lose too much water through evaporation, the skin becomes brittle and dry. Make sure your skin receives the replenishment it needs by drinking at least eight 8-ounce glasses of water every day.

Exercise

Exercise promotes good circulation, which ensures that your blood will be carrying oxygen and other nutrients to your skin cells, and the increased blood supply to the skin will make your complexion look rosier.

Use gentle cleansers

Avoid soaps that contain antiseptics and perfumes that may irritate and dry the skin and opt for those with fewer and more natural ingredients.

Limit the amount of time you spend in the bath

Surprisingly enough, water, especially hot water, can actually work to dry your skin by washing away the natural oils that help trap moisture in the skin. Try to get by on a quick shower or limit yourself to a ten to fifteen minute warm bath. If you long to soak in a hot tub, be sure to add bath oil to the water and apply moisturizer all over your body immediately after bathing.

Moisturize at least twice a day

A moisturizer works something like a protective shield, allowing the outer layer of your skin to build up natural moisture and keep the skin cells hydrated. Although department and specialty stores are filled with miracle moisturizers that promise to reverse the effects of aging, a moisturizer can only help to make the skin feel smooth, temporarily prevent moisture loss from skin cells, and decrease the fine lines caused by dryness. Don't be fooled into paying a high price for creams that contain collagen, protein, and hormones; these substances are ineffective as topical agents and provide no special benefits to the skin. Therefore, the most effective emollients are also the least expensive ones and include—among many others—petroleum jelly, mineral oil, lanolin, and cocoa butter. In general, the simpler the moisturizer, the better.

Unfortunately, no matter how well you care for your skin, it will nevertheless become dryer, less supple, and more wrinkled the older you get. For those of us who choose to partake, however, there are a number of chemical agents and surgical procedures that may help to repair some of the damage time has wrought on our skin.

HOT FLASH!
Liver Spots and the Sun

Despite their common monikers, liver spots—also known as old age spots—are not caused by either liver disease or by the aging process. Instead, the brown spots commonly found on the face, hands, and arms of older men and women result from long-term exposure to sunlight. To avoid such unsightly spots, cover all body parts exposed to the sun with sunscreen. If spots have already appeared, talk to your doctor about treating them with Retin-A, a vitamin A derivative that may help fade them away in just a few months.

Retin-A

A vitamin A derivative called tretinoin, first approved by the FDA as a treatment for severe acne, has proven to smooth out wrinkles and reduce blotchiness in some people. Marketed under the name Retin-A and available only by prescription, this preparation appears to work best on fine wrinkles and generally healthy skin, while doing little to affect deep wrinkles or very coarse skin. In addition, Retin-A causes skin inflammation in many people who use it. You should only use Retin-A under the directions of a physician or dermatologist who has experience with its use.

Dermabrasion and chemical peels

Both of these procedures involve removing the outer layers of skin, thereby reducing fine wrinkles such as crow's feet, scar tissue, skin discoloration, and many other surface blemishes. Dermabrasion uses a skin tool that actually "sands" down the skin's top layers. The process takes about thirty to sixty minutes and requires local anesthesia. It leaves the skin feeling raw and looking rather pink, but the healing process takes only about seven to fourteen days.

Chemical peels, on the other hand, involve coating the skin with a mild acid that works to gently "burn off" the surface layer. Generally speaking, chemical peels are more uncomfortable than dermabrasions and take several weeks longer for the skin to heal.

Collagen injections

As you may remember from Chapter Two, the protein called collagen is the chief component of skin and connective tissue. When injected into the dermis (the middle layer of skin), collagen can plump up the skin, thereby erasing fine wrinkles and scars. Although largely successful and having minimal side effects, collagen injections are both expensive and short-lived; the injected collagen breaks down within one or two years and must be reapplied to be effective.

Cosmetic surgery

Every day, thousands of women opt for cosmetic surgery to smooth out wrinkles, tighten sagging skin, and remove deposits of fat from their faces and bodies. As plastic surgeons come under closer scrutiny by their respective medical boards and by the media, cosmetic surgery is becoming safer and more reliable every day. If performed properly, cosmetic surgery provides many women with just the "lift" they need to make it through what can be a difficult aging process. If you can afford it and if it would add to your self-esteem and vitality, by all means talk the matter over with your physician and ask him or her to recommend you to a reputable, board-certified plastic surgeon.

However, you must be aware that cosmetic surgery involves serious risks that should be balanced against potential benefits. According to the American Society of Plastic and Reconstructive Surgeons, cosmetic surgery overall carries the same 2 percent rate of serious complications—such as infections and anesthesia-related deaths—as most major surgical procedures. In addition, each operation carries its own risks of unpleasant, often permanent side effects. Make sure you have all the facts before opting for plastic surgery of any kind.

SLEEP DISTURBANCES

At menopause, many women who never before have had trouble falling asleep find themselves plagued with insomnia. One reason for this sudden sleeplessness is that the hypothalamus, which is integral to the female sex hormone cycle, is also responsible for setting our sleep patterns. When the levels of estrogen and progesterone begin to fluctuate, the hypothalamus sends out irregular and upsetting signals that keep us awake. Moreover, many menopausal women are plagued with night sweats, the nocturnal version of hot flashes, which wake them up from a sound sleep with their hearts racing and their bodies drenched with heavy perspiration. To make matters worse, the emotional issues related to menopause—including concerns about our changing body image, fears about growing old, perhaps even worries about our financial future—often interfere with our ability to get a good night's sleep.

Although it is true that we tend to need less sleep as we age, if you feel yourself dragging during the day or tossing and turning during the night, it's important that you try to pinpoint the cause of your sleep disturbances and then to find a solution. Without enough rest, you're bound to become run down, irritable, and perhaps even physically ill.

If you suffer from night sweats and are unable to take estrogen to alleviate them, it's important that you make yourself as comfortable as possible. First, make sure your night-clothes and bed linens are made of cotton, which tend not to trap the heat your body produces during the night; as you may remember, rising body temperatures often trigger hot flashes. In addition, have an extra set of nightclothes next to your bed, so that you can change quickly should you become drenched with perspiration during the night. If you sweat excessively, you may want to keep an extra set of sheets available as well so that your linens are fresh and comfortable at all times. Some women find it helpful to make up the bed with double layers of sheets. That way, should the top layer become damp, it can be quickly and easily removed without creating the need to com-pletely remake the bed.

If night sweats aren't the culprit, review your daily and bedtime routines carefully and follow these simple tips for a better night's sleep:

Drink a glass of warm milk

Sometimes the oldest cures are the most effective. If you can't seem to fall asleep, try drinking a glass of warm milk about a half hour before going to bed. Milk includes high dosages of tryptophan, an amino acid believed to mediate estrogen's affect on the hypothalamus.

BEST BET!
If You Can't Sleep, Try Tuna!

Long prescribed as a sleep aid, a hot glass of milk is loaded with tryptophan, an amino acid that stimulates the production of a brain chemical known for its soothing effects. For millions of Americans who are either lactose intolerant or simply dislike milk, this cure-all simply won't do the trick. Luckily for those people, tryptophan is found in many other substances including beef, poultry, tuna, spinach, and eggs. So if you can't seem to get to sleep, a tuna sandwich just may be your ticket to dreamland.

Exercise regularly

Physical activity both reduces stress and relaxes your muscles. Try not to exercise in the evening, however, when activity may act as a stimulant.

Stay away from stimulants

Coffee, tea, chocolate, and cola products should be avoided, especially during the evening hours, because they all contain caffeine, a powerful stimulant.

Establish a regular sleeping schedule

Try to go to bed and get up at specific, set times every day and night. Most importantly, get up at the same time every morning, even if you've had a bad night's sleep, and stay up until the proper time for bed. Even if you have to drag yourself through one or two days, it's likely you'll eventually be tired enough to sleep fully and deeply through the night on a normal schedule.

Only use your bed for sleep (or for sex!)

If you begin to associate the bedroom with reading, watching television, or other active endeavors, you may be stimulated rather than relaxed when you jump in the sack. If you find yourself unable to sleep after relaxing for fifteen minutes or more after climbing into bed, get up and go into another room. Return only when you're sleepy. That way, you'll never associate the bed with anxiety about *not* sleeping, which can only set a vicious cycle of insomnia in motion.

Leave your worries outside the bedroom door

Although easier said than done, it is important to relax not only your body but your mind if you intend to get a good night's sleep. Many people find it helpful to write down their worries in a journal every night before they get into bed, thereby "exorcising" them from conscious thought.

SMOKING

Why would a book on menopause need to discuss the dangers of smoking cigarettes? Because it is the single most important risk factor for cardiovascular disease and many types of cancer, as well as a contributing factor in osteoporosis, early menopause, glaucoma, and several other conditions. About 35 percent of all smokers die prematurely of a smoking-related disease. Smokers are three times more likely to die of cancer than nonsmokers. The Framingham Heart Study found that men who smoke have a ten-fold increase from sudden death from cardiac arrest. Among women smokers, the mortality rate is fivefold over women non-smokers; in fact, in the last decade, lung cancer has surpassed breast cancer as the leading cause of cancer death in women.

Although you might think that the highly publicized dangers of smoking would be enough to make everyone who smokes snuff out her last cigarette once and for all, if you smoke you're not alone. According to the American Heart Association, nearly fifty million people in the United States still smoke cigarettes on a daily basis. Part of the reason so many people still smoke is that cigarette smoking is one of the most addictive habits known to man or woman.

In a 1988 report, the Surgeon General concluded that not only is nicotine—the primary ingredient in cigarettes—addictive, but it's addictive in the same way as other narcotics, like heroin and cocaine, are addictive. People who smoke become more and more tolerant to the effects of nicotine, needing more and more cigarettes to satisfy their craving for the drug. If they quit smoking, they experience similar withdrawal symptoms— nausea, fatigue, anxiety, insomnia, irritability.

It is a fact that up to 70 percent of all those who quit will at one time or another relapse and begin smoking again. But that's not to say that quitting is impossible. Studies have shown that 95 percent of all people who quit smoking do it on their own, going "cold turkey," so to speak.

Although nicotine is the most addictive substance in cigarettes, it is hardly the most toxic. Tar, for instance, is one of the most carcinogenic substances known. This fact has prompted researchers to find a way to feed the nicotine habit while removing the other harmful substances. Nicotine pills and gums, for instance, feed the smoker trying to quit small doses of nicotine so that he or she won't feel the need to light up a cigarette.

The newest nicotine replacement method is called the nicotine patch. Applied once a day on the arm or stomach of a reformed smoker, the patch secretes a small dose of nicotine into the bloodstream on a steady basis throughout the day. Without having to cope with what can be severe withdrawal symptoms from lack of nicotine, the patch-wearer can instead concentrate on breaking other smoking-related habits, like the need to hold a cigarette in the hand or mouth.

If you'd like to quit smoking, talk to your doctor about the patch. In addition, both the American Heart Association and the American Cancer Society have drawn up plans to help those who want to quit find the will power and the strength to do so. (See Appendix II: Resources.)

URINARY INCONTINENCE

As described above under "Sexual changes," the muscles and tissues in the pelvic area often become weak and stretched after menopause. For some women, this results in a condition known as stress incontinence, or the involuntary release of urine with only the mildest of stimuli. Much to their embarrassment, women affected by stress incontinence release urine when they laugh, sneeze, cough, lift a heavy object, or exercise.

Another source of urinary incontinence results from a condition known as pelvic prolapse, which occurs when the pelvic muscles that hold the organs in place become so stretched that a gap is produced. This gap allows the various organs to protrude into the vaginal wall. When the urethra, the tube that connects the bladder to the urinary opening, prolapses—a condition known as urethrocele—poor bladder control is often the result. Cystocele occurs when the bladder sinks into the vaginal canal, making the process of emptying the bladder more difficult. Hence, women with cystocele often feel the need to constantly urinate, even when they have just been to the bathroom. In addition, cystocele is the cause of many urinary tract infections (see below). A dropped, or prolapsed, uterus is another relatively common condition that may cause urinary dysfunction. When the muscles and ligaments that hold the uterus in place weaken and the uterus sags into the vaginal canal, it often pulls the bladder and urethra—as well as the rectum—down with it. As you might imagine, several types of urinary and bowel problems may result.

Estrogen therapy, although it may strengthen and thicken vaginal and urinary tract linings, cannot cure pelvic relaxation. In about 10 percent of prolapse cases, surgery to repair weakened walls and reposition the organs is necessary. In extremely rare cases of uterine prolapse, a hysterectomy to remove the organ is the only logical recourse.

However, since most cases of both stress incontinence and urinary incontinence due to pelvic relaxation are mild, most women can learn to cope on their own. Performing Kegel exercises (see above under "Sexual changes") on a regular basis will help keep the muscles that support the bladder, urethra, and rectum strong and well-toned. In the meantime, to avoid embarrassment, you may want to use a sanitary napkin to absorb any urine released unexpectedly.

URINARY TRACT AND VAGINAL INFECTIONS

Many menopausal women are plagued by frequent urinary tract and vaginal infections, which are both annoying and painful. Infections are more frequent at this time because the loss of estrogen has weakened the lining of the bladder, urethra, and vagina, making them more prone to injury and inflammation. In addition, low estrogen levels cause vaginal secretions to become less acidic and more alkaline, and thus more inviting to many harmful organisms.

To prevent infections from taking hold, it is important to keep your vagina and urinary tract as clean and healthy as possible without causing irritation or trauma. Follow these simple tips:

- Bathe your genitalia daily with a gentle, nonperfumed soap and water.
- Avoid hot baths, which can be drying. Opt instead for a warm bath laced with a gentle bath oil.
- Wear cotton underpants and pantyhose with cotton panties; synthetic fibers are known to trap moisture, air, and bacteria.
- Avoid the use of commercial douches or feminine

hygiene sprays. They are often drying and irritating, which increase the risk of infection.

- Take antibiotics—for any illness—only under careful physician supervision. Some antibiotics, particularly tetracycline, are known to upset the Ph balance of the vagina, making it more susceptible to harmful bacteria.

- Take vitamin C and B supplements if you are plagued with vaginal infections; many women find that they help control vaginal inflammation.

- Eat at least an 8-ounce container of active-culture yogurt every day. Yogurt contains certain bacteria known to de-activate harmful substances in the vagina. (An added benefit to yogurt treatment is the added calcium it provides.)

- Antifungal drugs once available only by prescription are now offered over-the-counter to women who suffer from chronic yeast infections. Once you've confirmed with your doctor that your bouts of itching, inflammation, or discharge are caused by fungus, feel free to use these inexpensive and effective preparations.

- Your body's ability to fight off both major and minor infections depends to a large extent on how you treat it. To keep your immune system ready and able to defend against environmental and internal invaders, get plenty of rest, exercise regularly, and eat a balanced diet.

As you've probably noticed, most, if not all, of the symptoms and side effects of menopause are affected by the foods we eat and the amount of exercise we receive. In the following two chapters, you'll learn how to design an eating plan and fitness regimen that will help you live the rest of your life with vigor, energy, and health—with or without estrogen.

CHAPTER 7

EATING RIGHT FOR A LONG, HEALTHY LIFE

More than twenty-five hundred years ago, the Greek physician and philosopher Hippocrates declared, "Thy food be thy remedy." Today, as we approach the twenty-first century, these words ring with particular urgency and truth. Every day, the connection between what we eat and the state of our health becomes more clear and well-defined.

With that said, we need only look at a few statistics to understand that the issue of food and eating is not so simple for most people. According to several recent studies, including one presented at a 1992 National Institutes of Health conference on diet and health, more than 63 percent of American adults are over the recommended weight range for their build. These women and men are unable to balance their bodies' actual need for food with the amount and type of food they eat on a day-to-day basis. The resulting obesity puts them at greater risk for a host of diseases, including atherosclerosis, breast cancer, diabetes, heart disease, and hypertension, among others.

Dietary imbalances and deficiencies are linked to many other serious health problems in addition to obesity: calcium depletion often results in osteoporosis; a diet high in fat and low in fiber is linked to colon and other cancers of the digestive tract; and excess sodium may lead to the development of hypertension, to name just a few diet-related conditions.

Clearly, a balanced diet—one that provides you with the nutrients you need without overdosing you with fat and extra calories—is crucial to your overall health and well-being. In this chapter, we'll work together to discover just what a balanced diet really is and how best to fit the foods you need into your diet every day.

THE CHANGING NEEDS OF THE MENOPAUSAL WOMAN

Your body is in a constant state of transition and regeneration. Every day, some of your cells die and others are created to replace them. Every day, millions of major and minor miracles—the steady beating of your heart, the digestion of food, the appreciation of taste, smell, and touch—take place within the chemistry lab that is your body. The catalyst for these processes? The nutrients in the food you eat every day.

At different times in your life, your body requires special ingredients to properly perform its many functions. When you are pregnant or breastfeeding, you need to consume more calories and nutrients than you do when you only have your own body to feed. If you pass through a period of relative inactivity—while recuperating from a broken bone, for instance—you may require fewer calories than usual but more calcium and vitamin C to help your body rebuild the bone.

As you age, your body also needs special attention, particularly after the menopause. Your metabolism—the rate at which food is used by the body—slows down and you will need to consume fewer calories to maintain your weight. In fact, in order to stay fit and trim, you may have to decrease your daily food intake by as much as 20 percent. The only alternative is to increase the amount of calories you burn every day by stepping up your activity level. Unfortunately, this slow-down in metabolism comes at a time when you might be exercising less often, thereby compounding the problem of weight gain. To offset these changes, you must either exercise more or eat less.

Maintaining bone strength and health is another priority when considering the changing dietary needs of the menopausal woman. As you lose estrogen, your bones require more calcium in order to regenerate themselves. To feed your bones, then, you'll need to eat more calcium-rich foods and/or take a calcium supplement (see below under "Vitamins and Minerals").

After decades of pumping gallons of blood, oxygen, and nutrients to every cell in your body, your heart and vascular system also demand extra special care if they are to continue to function well in your later years. The loss of estrogen, which is known to influence fat metabolism, speeds up the process of cardiovascular aging and disease in women. With or without estrogen, you should seek to lower your intake of fats as you get older.

No matter how well you care for your body, it will, eventually, be unable to perform its physiological miracles and will succumb to disease or simply give out. However, the time that it takes for our bodies to wear down has just about doubled in the past two hundred years. And, even more exciting, it appears that those extra years can be lived with health and vitality—if we pay careful attention to what we eat.

ESSENTIAL NUTRIENTS FOR A BALANCED DIET

The human laboratory requires about forty different essential nutrients in order to carry out bodily functions and maintain the body's health. These nutrients include oxygen, water, protein, carbohydrates, fats, and a host of vitamins and minerals. The body receives oxygen from the air you breathe; without it, you could not survive for more than a few minutes. Although most of us take oxygen for granted, study after study proves that the more oxygen you supply to your body's cells—by breathing deeply and circulating more oxygen-rich blood during aerobic exercise—the better.

Water, which is found in most everything we eat and drink, is another substance we tend to take for granted. Water regulates body temperature, circulation, and excretion, and aids in digestion. It bathes virtually all of our cells in moisture, and it is especially vital to the health and beauty of skin tissue. Nevertheless, few of us drink the 64 ounces of water our body needs every day to stay healthy.

The other thirty-eight or so essential nutrients are found in the food we eat. What we call a "balanced" diet is one that contains the appropriate amount—not too little and not too much—of those nutrients on a daily basis. In addition, a balanced diet also involves providing the right amount of calories—the energy value of food—to maintain proper body weight. A calorie represents the amount of energy the body would need to burn in order to use up that bit of food; any excess energy is stored as fat.

An average woman—moderately active, five feet four inches tall, 130 pounds, and about thirty-five years of age—burns approximately 1,755 calories every day. That means if she eats less than 1,755 calories (or exercises to burn more calories), she will end up using energy that has been stored as fat to make up the difference. On the other hand, if she eats *more* than 1,755 calories a day, she will end up gaining weight as excess glucose is stored in fat cells. One pound of body fat represents the consumption of about 3,500 extra calories.

As this thirty-five-year-old woman ages, she will find that her metabolism will begin to slow down just a bit every year, a rate that will accelerate after she passes through menopause. By the time she is sixty, for instance, she may burn just 1600 calories every day. Although she eats the same amount of food and exercises at the same level, she now stores an extra 155 calories every day. At this rate, she'll gain a pound in just under a month. Only by balancing her slower metabolism with either extra exercise or a modified—but balanced—diet, will she be able to avoid the dreaded middle-aged spread.

Most of us grew up with the idea that a balanced diet included equal amounts of four food groups: dairy, grains, meats, and fruits/vegetables. Today we know that eating right is a little more complicated than that. In fact, there are six different types of food—carbohydrates, fruits, vegetables, dairy, protein, and fats—and we need to eat each of those six foods in very different proportions because each contains different amounts of nutrients and calories.

Carbohydrates should make up the bulk of a nutritious diet. Fat, on the other hand, should form a very small portion of your day's diet. Proteins, dairy products, and fruits and vegetables are to be eaten in varying proportions. The actual quantity of food you'll want to eat will depend on how many calories you, as an individual, burn on a daily basis, but the *proportions* of each type of food remain the same for everyone. Carbohydrates, for instance, should make up about 55 to 60 percent of your daily intake, no matter how many calories that entails.

The purpose of any eating plan is to provide the human body with the essential nutrients it needs to survive. It goes far beyond the scope of this book to determine your personal caloric and/or nutritional needs, but there are literally hundreds of books, healthy eating plans (such as those offered by Weight Watchers and the American Heart Association), and qualified nutritionists available to help you (see Appendix II: Resources). In the meantime, let's take a look at those dietary elements of special interest to menopausal women.

DAIRY PRODUCTS

One of the most important components of an American woman's diet is also one of the most neglected. Not only do milk and milk products such as cheese and yogurt comprise our major source of calcium—which is essential to the health of our bones, especially as we get older—but also are good sources of protein, carbohydrates, vitamins, and minerals. Although adults require just two servings—about 2 cups of milk or 2 ounces of cheese—every day, most of us neglect this aspect of our diet. Some of us refrain from consuming enough dairy products because we fear their naturally high caloric and fat content, others because we cannot digest them properly.

It is true that whole milk and particularly whole milk cheeses contain a great deal of fat. One 8-ounce glass of whole milk contains 150 calories, nearly 50 percent of which are derived from fat. And just 1 ounce of cheddar cheese packs 119 calories, of which fat comprises about 71 percent. Luckily, however, there are low-fat alternatives that are both delicious and nutritious. An 8-ounce glass of skim milk, for instance, contains 90 calories of which just 6 percent come from fat.

Some people averse to milk are lactose intolerant, or unable to digest milk properly. The inability to digest milk occurs because the enzyme lactase, which breaks down the milk's lactose (milk sugar) in the intestines, is produced in abnormally small quantities. Many people who are lactose intolerant, however, are able to tolerate fermented milk products, such as buttermilk or yogurt, since some of the lactose is already broken down by the bacterial cultures in these products. In addition, many dairy companies now produce milk already treated with the enzyme lactase to aid in the digestive process.

If you find yourself unable to consume the recommended daily portion of dairy products, you must substitute other foods rich in calcium in order to preserve your health and your bones. Later on in this chapter, you'll read more about calcium, calcium-rich foods, and the potential benefits of calcium substitutes.

FAT

Fat has been proclaimed the great American enemy and largely for good reason. Americans, who have among the highest rates of cardiovascular disease in the world, also have one of the fattiest diets in the world. About 40 to 45 percent of all calories consumed today come from fats and usually from animal products rather than from plant sources, which would also contain complex carbohydrates.

If you're like most American women, you need to reduce the amount and type of fat in your diet. By doing so, you'll kill many birds with one dietary stone. First, by reducing fat you'll automatically reduce calories, helping you lose weight if you need to or maintain your weight at a time when your metabolism may be slowing down. Second, and just as important, lowering your daily intake of fat will help you guard against the development of atherosclerosis and heart disease. Keep in mind that, even if you're not overweight, you may still be consuming too much cholesterol and fat, which then circulates through the bloodstream, damaging vessels along the way.

Fat is actually one component of a broad category of substances called *lipids*. Lipids include fats, fatty acids, sterols, and other compounds that are not soluble in water. Although not all lipids are fats, the terms are often used interchangeably. Cholesterol (see below) is often categorized as fat, when actually it is a lipid.

With all the dire warnings about fat consumption, it may come as a surprise to learn that you do need to eat some fat—

about one tablespoon—every day to provide your body with essential fatty acids. Essential fatty acids are the raw materials for several vital body functions, including proper growth and blood pressure control, among others.

Basically, there are three different kinds of dietary fat, each with its own distinct properties:

- Saturated fats include animal products such as whole milk, some cheeses, butter, meat, cream, and hydrogenated vegetable shortenings. One way to recognize a saturated fat is that it is solid at room temperature. Saturated fats are the fats to avoid; they tend to raise the level of cholesterol in the blood by 5 to 10 percent.
- Unsaturated fats, also called polyunsaturated fats, include sunflower oil, corn oil, soybean oil, sesame oil, and other liquid fats of vegetable origin. These fats seem to actually lower the amount of harmful cholesterol in our bodies.
- Monounsaturated fats, like peanut oil and olive oil, also remain liquid at room temperature. These fats do not change the amount of cholesterol or add to the amount of fat in the bloodstream, and have been found to lower serum cholesterol.

Most fatty foods contain a combination of saturated and unsaturated fat, but one usually predominates. Needless to say, the more you can stress unsaturated or monounsaturated fats in your diet, the better. The American Heart Association, as well as other major health organizations, recommend that less than 10 percent of your dietary fat come from saturated fat.

For further information about how to cut cholesterol out of your diet, contact the American Heart Association and ask for a copy of its Prudent Diet for a Healthy Heart (See Appendix II: Resources).

CHOLESTEROL

Cholesterol is a lipid found mostly in animal products like egg yolks, animal fats, cream, and cheese, although other foods, such as avocados and certain shellfish, may also contain high quantities of the substance. Although cholesterol, like fat, is essential for a number of vital body processes including nerve function and cell reproduction, there is no need for anyone to consume any cholesterol at all; the body manufactures all it needs. The average American, however, consumes anywhere from 600 to 1500 mg of cholesterol each day, which is from two to five times the 300 mg limit most physicians recommend.

As discussed in Chapter Two, cholesterol comes in three forms: low-density lipoproteins (LDL) which carry lipids into the blood, high density lipoproteins (HDL) which tend to carry lipids out of the bloodstream, and very low density lipoproteins (VLDL). (VLDL's part in the development of atherosclerosis is not yet known, but a high level of VLDL indicates that there is too much fat in the bloodstream.) We are born with about half of our cholesterol in the form of HDLs, but because the typical American diet is so high in saturated fats and cholesterol, we tend to replace HDLs with LDLs as we grow older.

Cholesterol is found in a wide variety of foods, and it is quite easy to consume far too much of it if you're not careful. One egg yolk, for instance, contains 250 to 275 mg of cholesterol; two eggs for breakfast means that you're already well over your limit of 300 mg for the day.

VITAMINS AND MINERALS

Vitamins and minerals are substances that your body requires to help regulate metabolic functions within cells. They are essential to life. Without enough vitamin D, for instance, children develop rickets, a serious, degenerative bone condition. Lack of the mineral iodine has been known to cause goiter and other thyroid disturbances. And, as we've already discussed at length in Chapter Three, calcium is essential for proper bone growth and maintenance.

Generally speaking, only very tiny amounts of vitamins and minerals are required to carry out the body's metabolic functions (see Table 3, page 148). If you eat a balanced diet, you should receive all the nutrients you need from the food you eat. Contrary to popular belief, taking more vitamins and minerals than your body requires—in the form of supplements or from the diet—will not provide you with any extra health benefits. In fact, an overdose of nutrients can result in conditions just as serious those caused by a vitamin or mineral deficiency.

TABLE 3

Important Vitamins and Minerals: Their Sources and Daily Requirements

The body needs some forty different vitamins and minerals to flourish and function properly. Many of these nutrients must come from the foods we eat. Listed below are a few of the more important nutrients, the U.S.D.A.'s recommended daily allowances for each, and what foods contain them in quantity.

Nutrient	RDA	Food Source
Vitamin A	800 RE	Whole milk, butter, eggs, green leafy and yellow vegetables, liver, fish, apricots
Vitamin C	60 mg	Citrus fruits, strawberries, tomatoes, green leafy vegetables
Vitamin D	5 to 10 mcg	Fortified milk, fish, liver, egg yolks, butter
Vitamin E oils,	8 mg	Nuts, wheat germ, vegetable whole grain cereals, olives, spinach
Folic Acid	400 mcg	Green leafy vegetables, liver, wheat germ, legumes
Calcium	1,500 mg	Milk and milk products, green leafy vegetables, shellfish, citrus fruits, sardines
Potassium	no RDA (@ 1,875 to 5,625 mg)	Bananas, dried fruits, peanut butter, oranges, yogurt, dried peas and beans
Sodium	no RDA (less than 3,300)	Table salt, baking soda, processed foods, eggs, milk, poultry, fish, meat
Iron	10 to 18 mg	Liver, kidneys, egg yolks, peas, beans, nuts, raisins, enriched breads and cereals

That said, a recent spate of studies from across the United States and around the world has focussed on the anti-oxidant properties of certain vitamins, particularly vitamins C, E, and betacarotene (precursor of vitamin A). Anti-oxidants destroy certain molecules in the body called free radicals, which are known to contribute to many diseases, including heart disease and many types of cancer. It takes oxidation by a free radical to turn cholesterol into LDL, the "bad" cholesterol, for instance. Vitamins known to contain anti-oxidants appear to deactivate free radicals and thus help prevent buildup of LDL and the subsequent development of atherosclerosis.

One study on the role of anti-oxidants on heart disease was reported by Joann Manson, M.D., and Charles Hennekens, M.D., of Harvard Medical School and Brigham and Women's Hospital in Boston. After monitoring the diet and vitamin use of eighty-seven thousand nurses for more than a decade, the investigators found that the women whose vitamin E consumption was in the upper 20 percent had a 35 percent lower risk of heart disease, even when all other factors, like smoking, blood pressure, and cholesterol were taken into account. Those whose beta carotene consumption was in the upper 20 percent had a 22 percent lower risk of heart disease.

Does this mean we should all take mega-doses of vitamins? No—or at least not yet. The studies, although promising, are far from conclusive. No doctor—not even Dr. Hennekens who headed the study at Brigham & Women's—is about to recommend that you risk an overdose or waste your money on a measure that may or may not prove to be successful in the long run. To quote Dr. Hennekens from a September 22, 1992 article in the *New York Times*, "We ought to [prescribe vitamin therapy] only on the basis of reliable data from controlled trials."

Until that time, you should try to get your vitamins and minerals the healthy and natural way—by eating a healthful diet—and remain within the guidelines set by the Food and Nutrition Board of the United States government. (The Food and Nutrition Board is responsible for recommending the appropriate amounts of nutrients we should consume on a daily basis. These Recommended Daily Allowances (RDAs) are used by most nutritionists in setting guidelines for a healthy diet.)

There are a few exceptions, however. In general, vitamin intake should be increased if you are pregnant or breastfeeding. In fact, pregnant women should take about 15 to 50 percent more of most vitamins—and up to 100 percent more of vitamin D—than the general population. Since it may be difficult to receive those extra vitamins from diet alone, many physicians recommend vitamin supplements.

Of all the minerals required in our daily diets, only three present challenges to the general population, and especially to women: calcium, of which we tend to consume too little; sodium, of which we consume too much; and iron, which has recently become quite controversial. Let's discuss each of these minerals separately.

CALCIUM

Calcium is one of the most abundant and important minerals in the body. As you age, you need to consume extra calcium because your body no longer absorbs calcium from food as efficiently as it did when you were younger. In fact, the average adult absorbs just 15 percent of ingested calcium; the rest is excreted. In addition, the loss of estrogen inhibits the bone from efficiently using the calcium the body does absorb to rebuild itself.

Therefore, you need to consume more calcium after menopause simply to maintain the strength of your bones and your overall metabolic health. Although the RDA of calcium for women who aren't pregnant or breastfeeding is just 800 mg a day (the equivalent of about two and a half glasses of skim milk), the National Institutes of Health have recommend that menopausal women need as much as 1,500 mg of calcium, the equivalent of about five 8-ounce glasses of milk.

The best sources of calcium are dairy products, including milk, cheese, and yogurt (see Table 4, page 151). To avoid consuming too much fat, however, you should choose low-fat or skim versions of these products. For those of you who are lactose intolerant or simply do not enjoy dairy products, other foods may provide you with enough calcium as well. Sardines (with the bones) and leafy green vegetables, such as turnip greens and broccoli, are particularly good sources.

TABLE 4

Dietary Sources of Calcium

As women age, and especially after they lose estrogen at menopause, their need for calcium increases. The National Institutes of Health recommend that postmenopausal women consume at least 1,500 mg of calcium per day.

The best sources of calcium come from dairy products, but other foods contain high levels of the mineral as well.

Food	Portion	Calcium (mg)
Milk, whole or skim	8 oz	300
Yogurt, plain, whole	8 oz	275
Yogurt, skim with nonfat milk solids	8 oz	452
American cheese	1 oz	195
Cottage cheese	1 cup	211
Swiss cheese	1 oz	259
Mussels	3.5 oz	88
Salmon, canned/with bones	3.5 oz	100
Shrimp	3.5 oz	63
Sardines, with bones	3.5 oz	240
Almonds	1 oz	75
Sesame seeds	1 oz	28
Bean curd (tofu)	3.5 oz	128
Broccoli, cooked	1 cup	178
Collards, cooked	1 cup	150
Kale, cooked	1 cup	194

By far, the most efficient way to fulfill your calcium requirements is through the food you eat. Calcium works best in conjunction with other nutrients, like vitamin D, lactose, potassium, boron, and protein, that may be consumed along with the calcium-rich food. Milk, for instance, is almost always fortified with vitamin D and is also a good source of protein; both of these substances enhance the body's absorption of calcium.

However, if you find you are unable to meet your calcium needs through your diet, there are several different types of calcium supplements available. Generally, the least expensive and most widely available supplements are calcium carbonates and calcium lactate; both of these are absorbed by the body equally well but may cause gassiness and/or constipation among some users. A more expensive form of calcium, called calcium gluconate, tends to have fewer side effects. Several over-the-counter antacids, specifically Tums and Alka II, for example, contain about 200 mg of calcium per tablet. (Beware, however, that some antacids contain aluminum, which interferes with calcium absorption and should therefore be avoided.)

Foods and beverages fortified with a certain kind of calcium, calcium citrate malate, a supplement added to fruit juices, has proven to be quite effective. A 1990 Tufts University study reported that calcium citrate malate was more effective than calcium carbonate supplements in helping to reduce bone loss in the thigh, forearm, and spinal column.

It is important to note that not all calcium supplements are created equal: some are more difficult for the body to absorb than others and all contain different dosages of calcium. To choose which is best for you, consult first with your physician about your need for extra calcium and then with your pharmacist about which brand and type of supplement will be most effective for you.

SODIUM

Salt is another favorite staple of the American diet found to be anathema to overall good health. Excess sodium intake is related to high blood pressure, which is a major risk factor for heart attack and stroke. Although the actual physiological need for sodium may be as low as 220 mg a day, most Americans consume over ten times that amount, from 2,500 mg (or 2.5 grams) and up each day.

Sodium is a metallic element, active in the human body only when it occurs in combination with another element. Its most common form is table salt or sodium chloride (NaCl). In that form, it is used as a spice and as a preservative and is found in greater or lesser amounts in nearly everything we eat.

The main health hazard related to excess sodium intake is high blood pressure. If you consume too much salt and your kidneys are unable to excrete it, the level of fluids in your body will rise. This causes blood pressure to rise, since the vessels and heart must work that much harder to circulate the extra fluid.

Sodium does not cause high blood pressure in all individuals, however. There appears to be a segment of the population that is "salt sensitive," or genetically prone to high blood pressure caused by sodium retention. Nevertheless, an overdose of sodium, even among those of us not at risk for hypertension, should be avoided.

IRON

All cells in the body contain iron, which plays a vital role in many biochemical reactions. It is an especially crucial element in hemoglobin, the oxygen-carrying protein that gives blood its red color, and in certain muscle tissue. If you do not provide your body with enough iron over a long period of time, you may develop anemia—the depletion of red blood cells—which results in both exhaustion and highly increased risks of serious infections.

Iron deficiencies are common in this country, especially among low-income families who eat diets low in protein-rich foods, which also provide the lioness's share of dietary iron. Menstruating and pregnant women in all income brackets are also susceptible to iron deficiencies; menstruating women because monthly blood losses increase iron needs and pregnant women because the fetus places an extra demand on the blood supply.

However, recent studies indicate that many more Americans may be suffering from iron *overdoses*. A 1989 study of fourteen thousand adults funded by the National Institutes of Health, for instance, found that men who had high blood levels of iron were 37 percent more likely to develop cancer of the colon, lung, and bladder than men with lower iron levels. And an even more recent study, published in the September, 1992 issue of *Circulation*, sent shock waves through the medical community.

About nineteen hundred men from eastern Finland were tested for ferritin, an iron-storing protein, in 1986, then followed for five years. At the end of that period, fifty-one had suffered heart attacks. Researchers discovered that those men who more than two hundred micrograms of ferritin per liter of blood—a normal level—were twice as likely to have heart attacks compared with men with levels below two hundred. The risk more than quadrupled, the study went on to say, in men who had both high LDL and iron levels.

Scientists believe that iron may well act as an oxidant in the blood, promoting a reaction between LDLs and oxygen that results in atherosclerosis and coronary artery disease. If so, the fact that heart disease increases dramatically among menopausal women may be traced in part to the fact that they no longer menstruate and thus retain more iron in their blood.

What does this mean to the average woman facing menopause? It means that unless you are suffering from excessive abnormal bleeding, you should not take iron supplements. Do not neglect to consume the daily requirement of iron (about 10 mg), but watch out that you don't overdose either. One way to ensure the proper balance is by eating a high carbohydrate, low-fat/low-protein diet. If you have any concerns about iron and your heart, talk them over with your physician.

A NOTE ABOUT ALCOHOL

To drink or not to drink is a question that has taken on new meaning of late. It appears that moderate alcohol consumption— one to two drinks a day—may actually prove to be beneficial to many men and women, especially as they age. Menopausal women may benefit from taking an occasional drink because alcohol appears to raise estrogen levels by interfering with liver function; in fact, a recent study conducted at the University of Pittsburgh demonstrated that consuming three to five drinks per week elevates estrogen levels among postmenopausal women enough to offer extra protection against heart disease.

Men also receive beneficial effects from moderate alcohol intake. This phenomenon has been nicknamed the "French paradox" because the health benefits of alcohol consumption were first noticed among the French, who have far lower mortality rates due to heart disease than do Americans while eating a diet equal or higher in fat levels. The difference between the American and French diets appears to be in the amount of alcohol—specifically red wine—the two cultures imbibe. Red wine apparently affects the cardiovascular system by working to increase the levels of HDL, the "good" cholesterol. By what mechanism this occurs is still not completely understood, but scientists believe that certain chemicals in alcohol, known as phenols, work as anti-oxidants to help metabolize lipids and more quickly remove them from the bloodstream.

However, these benefits must be carefully balanced with the known risks of alcohol. After tobacco, alcohol abuse is the leading cause of premature death in America and is associated with the loss of more than one hundred thousand lives annually. Alcohol is associated with about half of the fifty thousand fatalities that occur on the nation's highways. In terms of other health risks, the statistics are equally bleak. Some studies have shown that even moderate drinkers run an increased risk of breast cancer and heavy drinkers have high rates of liver disease and heart disease.

Certainly, then, if you are unable to handle alcohol physically or emotionally, have a family history of alcoholism, or simply don't like to drink, the risks of alcohol far outweigh the benefits, and you should not feel pressured to partake.

LOSING WEIGHT

So far, we've been talking about nutritional requirements and very little about calories. Eating any kind of food, including fruits and vegetables, can cause you to gain weight, if you eat more calories than you burn off. The number of calories needed by a specific individual to meet his or her energy needs depends on several factors, including age, weight, and level of exercise. In addition, it must be stressed that there appears to be a very strong heredity factor involved in obesity; some people are born with a tendency to gain weight and those individuals may need special help in devising an eating plan that allows them to lose weight safely.

For most of us, however, the extra pounds that creep on as we age may have more to do with our eating and exercise habits than with heredity. Although your metabolism does slow down a bit after menopause, it is still possible to maintain or even lose weight at any age. To do so, you must follow one simple rule: consume fewer calories than you expend on a daily basis.

There are a number of ways to calculate the number of calories you need to maintain your weight or to lose or gain weight. The general rule of thumb is that the average, relatively active adult of normal weight requires about twenty-five to thirty calories per kilogram (2.2 pounds) of ideal body weight per day, or about thirteen calories per pound, to maintain the same body weight.

To lose weight, that same active adult should consume no more than about ten calories per pound of ideal weight. A thirty-five-year-old, 130 pound woman who takes an exercise class three times a week (burning about 600 to 800 extra calories altogether) could consume about 1,200 calories a day, and she could still expect to lose about one to two pounds per week. As she gets older, of course, she will probably have to step up her activity level if she still wants to lose weight, since her metabolism will gradually slow down. (Nutritionists and physicians have determined that to lose weight safely, no fewer than 1,200 calories should be consumed by anyone, regardless of weight, age, or activity level.)

In addition, *what* you eat matters just as much as *how much* you eat. Indeed, all foods are not created equal: if two people eat the same amount of food in a day, but one person takes in 60 percent of her food in the form of complex carbohydrates while the other consumes her calories in the form of fat, the two will most likely end up with very different body shapes and weights.

Why? First, complex carbohydrates are used more efficiently than fat and are far less likely to be stored in adipose tissue. Experiments at the University of Massachusetts Medical School, for example, suggest that if you consume 100 excess carbohydrate calories, 23 of those calories will be used simply to process those foods, and thus only 77 of them will end up being stored as fat. But it appears that only 3 calories are burned in the processing and storing of 100 fat calories.

Second, and most importantly, a gram of fat provides more than twice the calories of a gram of carbohydrates; 9 calories as compared to 4. That's why one ounce of potato chips—processed in fat and totaling more than 160 calories—is more fattening than one ounce of baked potato, which contains about 30 calories and no fat at all.

The best way to diet is to eat relatively small portions of a wide variety of foods and expect to lose just 1 to 2 pounds a week. Fad diets that promise rapid weight loss and concentrate on eating just a few select foods are dangerous for many reasons. By concentrating solely on losing pounds and not on learning proper nutrition, you'll most likely fall back into the same kinds of bad eating habits that made you heavy in the first place once you've lost weight. This kind of seesaw effect is both dangerous and counterproductive; rapid weight loss puts an extraordinary strain on the cardiovascular system and also changes the body's metabolic rate, forever lowering the number of calories your body needs to maintain vital functions. That's why people find it difficult to lose weight again after crash dieting.

By adapting proper portion control, you can combine the food types to develop a safe, healthy, and effective eating plan to lose weight. The following adaptation of a plan recommended by the American Heart Association and followed by Weight Watchers as well as other diet support groups, replaces the often tedious struggle of calories and "dieting" by the more natural approach of portion control and food variety.

By following the following plan, you should be able to lose weight easily and without feeling hungry. If you have a weight problem, though, you know that hunger is often the last of a long list of reasons to eat: boredom, frustration, stress,

TABLE 5

Your Daily Food Plan for Healthy Weight Loss

The following portions of protein, carbohydrates, fruits, vegetables, breads, dairy products, and fat will provide you with about 1,300 calories per day. Depending on your age and weight, this may translate to a healthy weight loss of 1 to 2 pounds a week; if you weigh more than, say 150 to 160 pounds, you may want to increase the amount of food prescribed here as well as exercise; if you weigh less than 120 to 130, you may require vigorous exercise to speed your metabolism as well as burn extra calories.

• **4 to 6 ounces of protein**	(chicken, turkey, fish, lean beef, veal, pork, lamb, lentils, dried peas, sprouts and grains, nuts, egg whites as desired; but only two or three whole eggs per week)
• **Three 1/2-cup servings (or more) of fresh vegetables**	
• **Three servings of medium sized fruit**	
• **Four servings of bread/starches,**	each involving no more than 80 calories (bread, English muffins, pasta, cereal, potatoes, rice, popcorn)
• **Two 8-ounce servings of low-fat milk,**	yogurt, or cottage cheese; this includes hard cheeses, but no more than four 1-ounce servings per week
• **No more than 2 tablespoons of fats**	

depression, excitement, to be sociable, and simply because food tastes good are just a few of the non-hunger-related reasons for eating. Add to that list a genetic predisposition to obesity and the stage is set for many of us to grow up with weight problems.

For this reason, many nutritionists suggest maintaining a food diary. That way, you can keep track of not only how many calories you take in and the types of food you eat, but you can also note *why* you eat. Although we're not always aware of our motivations at the time, we can often discover patterns of eating behavior after a few weeks of monitoring our daily diets.

Does losing—even maintaining—proper weight doom you to diet for the rest of your life? Not if you exercise. Consider this statistic: the average active thin person in America today eats an average of 600 calories a day *more* than her overweight peer. Note, however, that the key word here is *active*. Simply put, the more calories you burn through exercise, the fewer you'll store as fat. In the next chapter, you'll learn the principals of safe, effective activity.

CHAPTER 8

EXERCISING FOR LIFE

It's official: leading a sedentary life may just make you sick. In the fall of 1992, the American Heart Association formally designated inactivity as one of the four top risk factors for the development of heart attacks and stroke. Along with high blood pressure, cigarette smoking, and high cholesterol, the lack of exercise is a contributing factor in cardiovascular disease, the nation's number one killer.

The news is not all grim, however. In fact, the flip side of the startling equation "inactivity=disease" is quite encouraging: "exercise=disease prevention." By exercising regularly you can significantly lower your risk of stroke, hypertension, and myriad diseases that are influenced by obesity, such as breast cancer and diabetes.

Although we've still got a long way to go—only about 40 percent of all Americans exercise with any frequency—more and more of us appear to be heeding this life-saving message. In 1990, the Centers for Disease Control reported that the annual death rate from heart disease dropped 6 percent in just one year and much of that improvement is due to better exercise habits being practiced throughout the country.

For a woman entering or past the age of menopause, exercising may be the single best thing she can do for her emotional and physical health. Exercise mitigates three of her most pressing health challenges: cardiovascular disease, osteoporosis, and weight gain. Whether or not she takes estrogen replacement, the active postmenopausal woman has a much better chance of keeping her heart healthy, her bones strong, and her body fit than her more sedentary sisters.

Many women find that exercise alleviates other menopausal symptoms, including annoying hot flashes. A recent study among postmenopausal women at Wayne State University showed that more than 50 percent of hot flash sufferers decreased the frequency and severity of their episodes by exercising on a regular basis. In addition, a menopausal woman who exercises will probably notice that her skin looks and feels younger as more blood is pumped into the tiny capillaries that feed the dermis. Improved circulation will also help her digestive system stay healthy and her immune system strong.

Without question, a major benefit of exercise to the menopausal woman is the effect it has on her brain and her emotional life. Like the skin, brain tissue is fed by thousands of tiny capillaries; the more blood coursing through them to feed the brain, the more mentally alert and emotionally satisfied a woman will feel. Part of the reason is that certain body chemicals called endorphins, known to dull pain and produce a mild euphoria, are released during vigorous exercise. Smokers who exercise find it easier to quit, therapists frequently prescribe exercise to their depressed patients, and dieters who also exercise claim to feel less hungry and more self-confident about meeting their weight loss goals than they did when they were sedentary.

Last, but hardly least, exercise will help the postmenopausal woman maintain her weight, or even lose weight, even as her metabolism slows as she ages. Not only will staying fit directly help her avoid developing serious diseases, such as diabetes and heart disease, but by exercising she will look and feel younger and more energetic. In fact, the National Institutes of Health refers to exercise as the "most effective anti-aging pill ever discovered."

TYPES OF EXERCISE

In essence, there are two basic types of exercise: aerobic and anaerobic. The purpose of aerobic exercise is to improve cardiovascular health by forcing the body to deliver ever larger amounts of oxygen to working muscles. In fact, the word aerobic is derived from a Greek word meaning "air." Anaerobic exercise, (exercise "without air") on the other hand, attempts to strengthen individual muscles, which draw on their own sources of energy and do not require the body to increase its supply of oxygen. Also known as muscle conditioning or weight training, anaerobic exercise tries to build muscle mass while keeping the body strong and flexible.

In recent years, the benefits of aerobic exercise on both the cardiovascular system and on weight loss efforts have been well-publicized—and the popularity of aerobic dance classes is certainly testimony to the success of that publicity. Indeed, the effects of aerobics, which uses large muscle groups to get your heart pumping and your lungs filling with oxygen, are substantial.

However, new studies indicate that combining aerobics with weight training may be the best way to achieve overall health and fitness. Muscle is more metabolically active than fat: the body must burn more calories to feed and nourish muscle tissue than it would to maintain fat. Therefore, the more muscle you have, the more calories you'll burn every day.

In one 1992 study, exercise physiologist Wayne L. Westcott, Ph.D., the national YMCA's strength-training consultant, compared men and women who did thirty minutes of aerobic activity three times a week with those who combined fifteen minutes of aerobics with fifteen minutes of weight training. Surprisingly, after just eight weeks, those who'd added weight training lost more than twice as much weight as those who only did aerobics: the aerobic exercisers lost about four pounds compared to the ten pounds of fat lost by the weight-training group. Equally important, the aerobic exercisers lost one half pound of muscle, while the weight trainers had a net gain of two pounds of muscle.

Later in this chapter, you'll learn more about each type of exercise and how to create a program of fitness that will help you stay strong and healthy. In the meantime, it's important to know that exercise and fitness need not be elaborate or demanding: a recent study at the USDA Human Nutrition Research Center on Aging at Tufts University showed that nonathletes who merely moved around a lot in their daily lives had less body fat than those who were more sedentary.

Indeed, simply being more *active* every day will do a lot to improve your overall health. Instead of taking the elevator, walk up three or four flights of stairs. Carry your own luggage instead of hiring a bellcap or porter on your next vacation. Look at your household and gardening chores as great chances to stretch, lift, and bend your body instead of mere drudgery. Most important of all, put away the keys to your car and use your feet instead. A study conducted at the Cooper Institute for Aerobics Research in Dallas showed that women who walked vigorously three miles a day, five times a week increased their cardiorespiratory fitness by 16 percent, a rate comparable to that achieved by running, aerobics classes, and other, more vigorous aerobic activities.

In short, get exercise any way that you can and the more exercise you get the better.

EXERCISE AND YOUR HEART

How does exercise improve cardiovascular health? One link is between exercise and weight reduction—the more you exercise, the more calories you burn, helping you to lose extra pounds. In addition, a number of studies have found that regular, vigorous exercise can both lower total blood cholesterol and increase the ratio of HDLs to LDLs. After following five hundred healthy middle-aged women for three years, for instance, researchers at the University of Pittsburgh found that women who burned just three hundred calories more per week than they did at the start of the study were able to maintain healthy levels of HDLs. As you know, this reduces the risk for atherosclerosis, a leading health problem among postmenopausal women.

The heart itself benefits from a good workout: because your muscles need more oxygen when they're at work, the heart must pump harder to get extra oxygen-rich blood to them. Normally, the heart pumps about six quarts of blood a minute in an average adult woman, but when the body is exercising, blood volume to and from the heart rises to about twenty-five quarts per minute. This extra work strengthens the heart muscle; the stronger it is, the less hard it has to work to meet the body's need for oxygen. Exercise helps improve the health of the entire circulatory system because it distributes blood more evenly to all the blood vessels, even to the tiniest capillaries.

To improve cardiovascular health, you should choose to perform aerobic exercise, which involves working large muscle groups (such as leg muscles), for a sustained length of time. With regular aerobic exercise, your heart will eventually be able to pump more blood, and your vessels will be able to deliver more oxygen to the cells throughout the body in a more efficient manner. Swimming, jogging, cycling, singles tennis, skiing, rowing, dancing—any of these activities, done regularly, will boost your heart rate and provide your body with all the benefits of exercise described above.

In order for aerobic exercise to have a healthy effect on the cardiovascular system, it must be of a sufficient intensity and frequency. You should exercise at a level of intensity called your target heart rate, or the rate at which your heart must work to provide health benefits to the cardiovascular system. At this rate, you will burn about three hundred calories in thirty minutes.

Target heart rates are calculated by using a simple formula. Your target heart rate is between 60 and 80 percent of your maximum heart rate; your maximum heart rate is calculated by subtracting your age from 220. The average fifty year old then would have a maximum heart rate of 220 − 50, or 170. Your target heart range should be from 102 to 136 beats per minute, which is 60 to 80 percent of your maximum heart rate. Average target heart rates for women forty years and above are listed below:

Training Heart Rates by Age

Age	60%	80%
40	108	144
45	105	140
50	102	136
55	99	132
60	96	128
65	93	124

You can determine whether or not you are within your target zone by taking your pulse immediately after exercise. The easiest way to take your pulse is to place two fingers (not your thumb—it is also a pulse point and can disturb the accuracy of your reading) on your wrist. Count the beats for ten seconds, then multiply that number by six. If your pulse rate is below the target range, you should increase either the intensity or the length of your workout. If your pulse is above your target rate, slow down.

In addition to being aerobic and intense, exercise must be performed on a regular basis. For cardiovascular benefits to be achieved, exercise should be done about three times a week, preferably at your target heart rate, for at least thirty minutes. Keep in mind that this is a goal to strive for; if you're not in shape, it will take some time for you to be able to exercise at this level.

EXERCISE AND YOUR BONES

A 1987 survey on exercise, diet, and bone loss in the *Journal of American Geriatrics Society* found that sedentary nursing home residents in their eighties experienced more than a 4 percent increase in density of the forearm bone when they performed mild exercises three times a week for three years. A group of nonexercisers underwent a 2.5 percent *decline* in bone density over the same period of time. That news should encourage all women who are approaching or past the age of menopause because osteoporosis is one of the most common and debilitating conditions related to the loss of estrogen.

Before we discuss the best bone-building exercises, it is important to stress that exercise alone will probably not repair extensive bone damage that has already taken place. However, taken together with estrogen replacement and calcium supplements, exercise may help you strengthen your bones or, at the very least, protect against future bone loss.

For exercise to be effective against osteoporosis, it must be what is known as *weight-bearing*: it must provide the stress of muscles pulling on bone, in effect adding to the force of gravity, which is why they are sometimes called "anti-gravitational exercises." (Astronauts who spend long periods of time in gravity-free environments develop osteoporosis quickly, because their bones are not being stressed by their muscles.) Weight-bearing exercises that work the long bones in the legs include walking, jogging, tennis, and other exercises that are also considered aerobic exercise, because they also work the cardiovascular system.

However, the effects of exercise on bone are limited: they only produce benefits in the exact bones that are stressed by the exercises. A right-handed tennis player, for instance, will have much denser, stronger bones in her right arm—the arm she stresses during the game—than in her left arm. Aerobic exercise, which usually focusses on the long bones of the legs, tends to be ineffective in preventing osteoporosis because it strengthens only the leg bones. The best way to protect against osteoporosis, then, is to add weight training and muscle conditioning exercises that work both your upper body muscles—including those of the back, arms, and stomach—as well as the lower body.

The purpose of muscle conditioning is to increase both the strength and endurance of your muscles by applying resistance to normal body motion, thereby making the muscles work harder (and placing more stress on the bones). Every time a muscle is worked in this way, it becomes a bit stronger and bigger.

Calisthenics, which are floor exercises like sit-ups, push-ups, and leg lifts, use the weight of your own body as resistance and are usually quite effective, especially for beginners. Free weights (otherwise known as barbells) and weight training with machines like Nautilus and Cybex allow you to increase the resistance gradually by adding weight as your muscles develop.

It is extremely important that muscle conditioning exercises are done properly—and that usually requires instruction and advice from an expert. Visit your local YWCA or join a health club to develop the best, and safest, weight-training program for you.

PLANNING AN EXERCISE PROGRAM

Your first step in developing an exercise program is to consult with your physician, especially if you're overweight, over forty, or have any other risk factors for cardiovascular disease. Your doctor may recommend that you take a stress test, which measures how your heart and blood vessels are functioning. A stress test involves nothing more than having your heart rate measured by EKG (electrocardiogram) and your blood pressure monitored by a technician while you jog on a treadmill or ride a stationary bicycle. One of the most important benefits of the stress test is that it helps diagnose heart and vessel disease through changes in the EKG tracings. It will also help determine the amount of exercise your heart and muscles can handle without any adverse effects. Both the length of time you are able to exercise and the intensity of activity you are able to endure without becoming exhausted will help your doctor determine a safe exercise routine for you.

Regardless of the type of exercise you choose, every session should contain three elements: 1) a warm-up; 2) an exercise phase (either cardiovascular or muscle conditioning or both); and 3) a cool-down. Ideally, the entire session should last about forty-five to sixty minutes.

1) A five to ten minute warm-up is essential to warm your muscles. Warming up prepares you for exercise by gradually increasing your heart rate, blood flow, and muscle action. Contrary to popular belief, however, a good warm up does not begin with stretching; stretching cold muscles can injure them. Instead, you should jog in place for a minute or two before you start to stretch.

2) The aerobic phase of the exercise should last approximately thirty minutes at your target heart rate. However, beginners who are out of shape may have trouble sustaining intense exercise for that long. Many experts suggest reducing this phase of the workout session to about five to ten minutes for a few weeks until your heart and muscles have gained some capacity and strength. If you decide to combine aerobics with weight training at the same time, it may be best to shorten your aerobic routine to perhaps twenty minutes.

3) A weight training and muscle conditioning routine should involve about thirty minutes of slow—but constant—stress on different muscles of the body. Your exact exercise routine should be formulated with an exercise specialist in a gym or at the YWCA, but generally speaking it consists of about a dozen exercises: six for the upper body and six for the lower body.

No matter what type of exercise program you choose, it is important that if you feel any of the following symptoms while exercising, *stop exercising immediately* and *consult your physician to determine the basis of the symptoms.* They could be signs of some cardiovascular stress, such as a heart attack or stroke:

- Chest discomfort, including pain, tightness, heaviness, or breathlessness
- Any discomfort or numbness in the jaw, neck, or arm
- Dizziness
- Headache
- Nausea

4) The third phase of your workout session is called the cool-down. It consists of two parts. First, gradually reduce the level of intensity of whatever activity you're performing. If you choose to jog, for instance, don't suddenly stop and sit down. Instead, walk a block or two at a somewhat slower pace. Then stretch gently for about five minutes. Cooling down will both help you avoid muscle stiffness and reduce the chances of an abrupt drop in blood pressure that can occur when exercise comes to a sudden halt.

KEYS TO MAINTAINING YOUR EXERCISE PROGRAM

You've checked with your doctor. You've started to exercise, and you've been keeping to a pretty regular schedule of three workouts per week. You know in your heart that your exercise program should last forever, that regular exercise must become a part of your daily life if lasting health benefits are to be derived. But you've seen others fail in their same very good intentions. Perhaps you've failed before, too.

To help you stick to an exercise routine, try one or more of these hints:

1) Choose activities you enjoy

Consider this: if you exercise for forty-five minutes three times a week for a year, you'll be spending 117 hours—the equivalent of about three full forty-hour work weeks—sweating and striving at one activity or another. The likelihood that you'll stick with such a routine depends to a large degree on enjoying what you're doing every time. Very often people start exercising with great enthusiasm, but after just a few weeks revert to their former sedentary ways. Boredom, inconvenience, and lack of motivation are all at the top of former exercisers' reasons for quitting. Finding an activity that excites or motivates you will help strengthen your resolve; so will altering your routine and adding new activities whenever you start to feel bored. Take a dance class one session, lift weights the next, bicycle outside a few days in a row, then play a game of tennis.

2) Set realistic goals

How many of us have vowed to transform ourselves into Christy Brinkley by logging in two hours a day every day at the gym? And how many of us, after missing just one session, have declared ourselves failures and have given up completely? After failing to meet an unrealistic goal, or straining our muscles trying to do so, we often become so frustrated we decide not to exercise at all. To avoid this self-defeating trap, set goals you know you can meet, or perhaps ones just slightly out of reach. Achieving them will give you a sense of pride and self-confidence sure to keep you motivated.

3) Set a personal, cosmetic goal

Is your stomach rounder than you'd like it to be? Are your thighs too heavy? Your upper arms too flabby? If you're like most women, there's one part of your body that you'd like to change more than any other. If it helps motivate you to exercise, then keep that body part in mind while you work out. For instance, if you'd like to flatten your stomach, try doing sit-ups at a relatively fast pace. You'll not only condition your stomach muscles, but you're also likely to get your heart pumping faster as well. Running or jogging will not only strengthen your heart, but will do wonders for conditioning your gluteus maximus— the muscles of the potentially sagging buttocks.

4) Seek convenience

Eliminate as many excuses as possible for not exercising. If you join a health club that is only open during hours you are at work, for instance, then obviously you're setting yourself up to fail. Scheduling times to exercise—and treating your exercise times as if they were business appointments—is often the only way to incorporate aerobic activity into your lifestyle.

5) Find a support group

For most of us, there comes a time when our motivation sags and we lose interest in exercising on a regular basis. When this happens—preferably *before* this happens—enlist a friend or loved one to join you in your quest for cardiovascular health. Often, a little competition and companionship go a long way.

Without doubt, exercising will help you to feel healthier, more energetic, and yes, even younger, as will eating right and following some of the tips outlined for you in Chapter Six. On the other hand, there's no getting around it: there's no cure for aging or for the natural changes that come with it. Every woman will pass through menopause at one time or another and—with or without taking HRT—she is bound to feel at least some physical discomfort and emotional turmoil during this transition. We hope that this book has given you the information you need to formulate a positive and successful strategy for meeting the challenges ahead.

APPENDIX I

THE TEN MOST IMPORTANT MEDICAL TESTS FOR MENOPAUSAL WOMEN

1. Blood cholesterol
2. Blood pressure
3. Blood sugar
4. Bone density
5. Breast exam, self
6. D & C
7. Endometrial biopsy
8. Mammography
9. Pap smear
10. Pelvic exam

CHOLESTEROL AND BLOOD LIPIDS

The amount of fats—also known as lipids or lipoproteins, of which cholesterol is a major component—circulating in your blood determines to a large degree your risk for developing atherosclerosis, a major risk factor for heart attacks and strokes. Estrogen apparently works to metabolize fats in a way that protects most women from developing atherosclerosis before menopause. If you decide not to take estrogen after menopause, your risks for cardiovascular disease increase dramatically.

Purpose

To measure the amount of lipids and fats circulating in your blood.

The test

A simple blood test, known as lipoprotein-cholesterol fractionation.

Special instructions/precautions

Prior to having the blood test, most physicians recommend that you:

- eat a normal diet for two weeks
- do not exercise for twelve to fourteen hours
- do not drink any alcohol for twenty-four hours
- inform the technician drawing the blood if you are taking any medications

What the test will show

The lipoprotein-cholesterol fractionation measures total blood cholesterol, low-density lipoprotein, high-density lipoprotein, and triglyceride levels circulating in the blood. See Best Bet! in Chapter 3, page 63, to determine proper levels.

When to schedule

Annually.

BLOOD PRESSURE

Today, an estimated sixty million Americans have high blood pressure, making it one of the nation's most widespread health problems. It is also one of our most serious: hypertension is the leading risk factor for heart attack and stroke, two of the three leading causes of death in the United States (along with cancer). As you age, your risks for this condition increase: one study conducted in 1985 showed that more than 50 percent of people over fifty-five years of age were hypertensive.

Purpose

To measure how hard the heart and vessels must work to nourish your cells with blood.

The test

Blood pressure is measured by an instrument called a sphygmomanometer. This instrument allows physicians to calculate how hard the heart is pumping and how much the blood vessels must contract to push the blood along. The first action is called systole, which means the contraction of the heart; the blood pressure is at its highest point during systole. When the heart is at rest, filling with blood, the blood pressure is at its lowest. We call this stage diastole.

Special instructions/precautions

Having your blood pressure taken is simple and absolutely painless. It involves rolling up your sleeve, having a blood pressure cuff wrapped around your upper arm, and allowing the doctor to listen through a stethoscope or watch a digital readout of the movement of your blood.

What the results will show

Your doctor will give you a number representing how hard your heart and vessels are working. A blood pressure of 120/80 is considered to be a perfect reading, but blood pressure will depend on your age, weight, and other factors. Also, if you are diabetic, you may need to keep your blood pressure even lower than other individuals since your blood vessels may be more fragile; speak with your physician. The Joint National Committee on Detection, Evaluation and Treatment of High Blood Pressure recommends that more than one, and preferably three, separate blood pressure reading be taken during a physical exam and an average reading calculated.

	DIASTOLIC	SYSTOLIC
NORMAL	85 or lower	140 or lower
HIGH NORMAL	85 to 89	
MILD	90 to 114	140 to 159
SEVERE	115 or higher	160 or higher

When to schedule

Annually, as part of your regular check-up. If you are prescribed an antihypertensive drug, you will need to be monitored more often and may want to consider a home testing kit for your convenience.

BLOOD SUGAR (GLUCOSE)

More than fourteen million Americans, most of them over the age of fifty, suffer from diabetes mellitus, an endocrine disorder in which your pancreas is unable to produce or use properly the hormone insulin, which is required to properly metabolize the food you eat. Although the symptoms are often so mild as to be unnoticeable, the high blood levels of sugar and fat that result are a major factor in the development of serious vessel disease affecting the heart, brain, kidneys, eyes, and lower extremities.

Purpose

To determine the concentrations of sugar in your blood or urine. Glucose in the urine is a condition called "glycosuria"; a high glucose concentration in the blood is termed "hyperglycemia."

The test

Most cases of diabetes mellitus are diagnosed from a blood test or urine test performed as part of a routine physical.

Special instructions/precautions

Often, there are no special instructions involved. However, your doctor may ask you to fast for eight hours before the blood test, or to eat two hours before the test, in order to more exactly gauge how well you metabolize food.

What the results will show

The blood and urine tests show the amount of glucose in your body. That amount is measured against the average, healthy amount for someone of your age, weight, and physical condition. If it is higher than normal, you may be given a diagnosis of diabetes. Treatment for diabetes includes diet, exercise, and, in some cases, medication with pills and/or injections of insulin—the hormone your body no longer uses properly.

When to schedule

Blood/urine sugar is usually measured every year during a regular check-up. However, if you suffer from excessive thirst and/or unexplained weight loss—the hallmark signs of diabetes—ask your doctor about the disease, especially if it runs in your family.

BONE DENSITY
Osteoporosis affects nearly half of all postmenopausal women and is responsible for more than seven hundred thousand bone fractures every year.

Purpose
To measure the thickness, width, and mineral content of bones.

The test
In essence, a sophisticated x-ray, photon absorptiometry emits a fraction of the radiation of conventional x-rays and is sensitive enough to detect a bone loss of just 1 to 3 percent. (Another more sophisticated and expensive technique, called quantitative digital radiology, is faster and more precise but is not yet in widespread use.)

Special instructions/precautions
You will lie still—usually fully clothed—while the scan is directed at either your lumbar region (spine) or on one of your hips. The entire test takes about five to seven minutes. Remember, however, that although the test takes a long time, it does not expose you to any dangerous level of radiation.

What the results will show
Your physician determines the health of your bones by assigning a numerical value to what he or she sees on the x-ray. Then your doctor places that number on a graph with the average bone density for someone of your age, height, weight, and ethnic background. If your number falls below that of the average woman of similar age and background, then you may be diagnosed with osteoporosis.

When to schedule
If you are at risk for osteoporosis or have suffered suspicious fractures after the age of fifty-five.

BREAST EXAM, SELF

Approximately one in nine American women will develop breast cancer in their lifetime. Early detection and treatment has been found to result in significantly better prognoses. In conjunction with regular mammograms (see page 179) after the age of forty, breast self-exams are every woman's responsibility.

Purpose

To detect lumps and changes in shape so that any problem can be diagnosed and treated as quickly as possible.

The test

Using your own hands, you will palpate your breasts in two positions, standing and lying down.

Special instructions/precautions

See diagram for directions. Perform the test at the same time every month, preferably a week after your period ends (if you are still fertile) or, if postmenopausal, the same day every month. By performing the exam regularly, you'll get to know how your breasts are supposed to feel—some of you may have naturally lumpy breasts, for instance—and therefore will be able to discern any *changes* in them. The changes in shape, tenderness, or lumpiness is what you'll want to report to your physician.

What the results will show

About 90 percent of all lumps discovered by self-exam or by mammography are benign. Breasts are extremely sensitive to hormonal changes; a lumpy, tender breast at any age could be due to stimulation by estrogen or other hormones. Fibroids (benign tumors), cysts, and infections of the milk glands are also common in postmenopausal women. Breast cancer will be ruled out through a biopsy—surgical removal of breast tissue.

When to schedule

Give yourself a self-exam once a month, preferably on the same day and time.

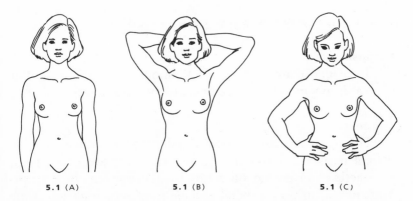

5.1 (A)   5.1 (B)   5.1 (C)

FIGURE 5.1 Breast self-exam. Stand in front of a mirror with arms at your sides. (A) Look for any changes, such as puckering or dimpling of the skin, discharge from the nipples, or a change in size of one or both breasts. Repeat examination first with arms overhead (B), then with arms on your hips and with your chest muscles tensed (C).

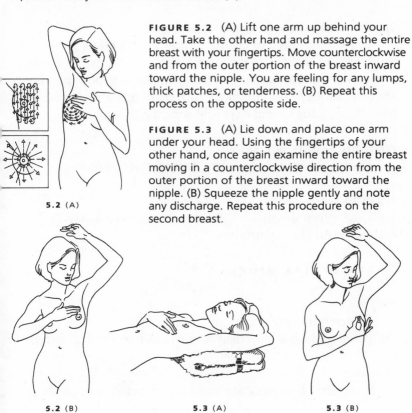

FIGURE 5.2 (A) Lift one arm up behind your head. Take the other hand and massage the entire breast with your fingertips. Move counterclockwise and from the outer portion of the breast inward toward the nipple. You are feeling for any lumps, thick patches, or tenderness. (B) Repeat this process on the opposite side.

FIGURE 5.3 (A) Lie down and place one arm under your head. Using the fingertips of your other hand, once again examine the entire breast moving in a counterclockwise direction from the outer portion of the breast inward toward the nipple. (B) Squeeze the nipple gently and note any discharge. Repeat this procedure on the second breast.

5.2 (A)

5.2 (B)   5.3 (A)   5.3 (B)

D & C (DILATION AND CURETTAGE)

Purpose

To diagnose any of several conditions of the uterus and/or to treat heavy menstrual bleeding and menstrual irregularities.

The test

The operation can be performed on an in-patient or out-patient basis at a hospital. You will require a local or general anesthetic. You lie flat on a table with your legs in stirrups. Your physician uses a metal speculum to open and widen the vaginal walls; a series of rods are used to dilate or stretch the cervix. Then a sharp, spoon-shaped instrument known as the curette is inserted and used to carefully scrape the uterine walls. The test takes about ten to fifteen minutes to perform.

Special instructions/precautions

You will be asked to fast for at least twelve hours prior to the procedure; to make sure the large intestine is empty, an enema is often given. In most cases, you'll stay in bed for about two hours after the surgery. You are likely to feel cramping and experience mild bleeding for several days following the procedure.

What the results will show

The results of the procedure depend on the purpose.

When to schedule

Your gynecologist will determine the need for a D & C, depending on your symptoms.

ENDOMETRIAL BIOPSY

Purpose

To determine the health of the endometrium—the lining of the uterus—which is extremely sensitive to hormonal stimulation.

The test

Endometrial biopsies are usually performed in your doctor's

office without an anesthetic. You will lie flat with your feet in stirrups while your doctor inserts a small instrument into the cervix and uterus to obtain a small sample of endometrial tissue.

Special instructions/precautions

The test takes only a minute or two and should not cause more than a momentary pinch of pain. You may experience mild cramping following the procedure.

What the results will show

The tissue removed from your uterus will be sent to a lab where it will be examined for the presence of abnormal cells. Its thickness and other effects of hormonal stimulation will be measured. If cancer is suspected, another type of biopsy and exam will be required.

When to schedule

Many physicians recommend this test prior to prescribing HRT. If you take estrogen without progesterone, an annual endometrial biopsy is recommended.

MAMMOGRAPHY

More than 135,000 women every year are diagnosed with breast cancer and 50 percent of breast cancers strike women between the ages of forty-five to sixty-five.

Purpose

Mammography can detect tumors so small that neither you nor your physician can feel them.

The test

A simple x-ray performed at a hospital or clinic. You will strip to the waist and wear a cotton drape. A technician will place one breast, then the other, under the x-ray machine. The entire procedure takes only a few minutes and is almost completely painless, although some women find the compression of the breast between the two x-ray plates uncomfortable.

Special instructions/precautions

Mammograms are not infallible; both false positives (diagnosis of a tumor when there is none) and false negatives (failure to detect a tumor) are common. But combined with regular self-exams and manual exams by your physician, mammograms are quite effective in detecting cancer early.

What the results will show

Any abnormal lumps or masses within the breast.

When to schedule

Unless you are at particularly high risk because of family or personal history, you do not need a mammogram until you are above age forty. From the ages of forty to forty-nine, women should have a mammogram every two years. After the age of fifty, most physicians recommend annual mammograms.

PAP SMEAR

Purpose

To detect cancerous, precancerous, and other abnormal cells (including urogenital viral infections and sexually transmitted diseases) on the cervix—the neck of the uterus that protrudes into the vagina.

The test

Performed as part of a routine pelvic exam, the pap smear involves the insertion of a speculum into the vagina and the wiping of a cotton swab or wooden spatula across the cervix. The smear is then transferred to a glass slide.

Special instructions/precautions

You should not be menstruating or have had sexual intercourse for twenty-four hours before the test.

What the results will show

Lab analysis will determine where within three categories your cervical cells fall: negative means you are fine; mild dysplasia means you have some infection and should be screened more regularly; and a positive test means there is a detectable change in the cells requiring further examination.

When to schedule
Every year as part of a routine pelvic exam or if cervical cancer is suspected.

PELVIC EXAM

Purpose
To check on the health of your pelvic organs by manual external and internal examination. A pelvic exam helps diagnose pregnancy, the cause of any irregular or unusual menstrual bleeding or pain, and serves as a general check before you are prescribed contraception or HRT.

The test
Your physician will use his or her hands to examine your pelvic organs. You will lie flat on your back with your knees bent (often your legs will be placed in stirrups). Your doctor will put one or two gloved fingers inside your vagina and the other hand on top of your abdomen to feel the size, shape, position, and tenderness of the uterus, ovaries, and fallopian tubes. Then your physician will place a speculum—a metal or plastic instrument—into the vagina to separate the walls of the vagina so the cervix can be examined. A visual examination is then made by the doctor with the aid of a tiny flashlight. At this time, a pap smear is usually taken.

Special instructions/precautions
The pressure placed on your stomach and internal organs by the doctor's fingers and hands may make you feel uncomfortable, but you should experience no pain. It is important to breathe normally and to try and stay relaxed during the exam, which should take about five minutes.

What the results will show

Your doctor will be able to tell quite a lot about the health of your pelvic organs through this exam, including whether fibroids, cysts, or infections are present.

When to schedule

Annually.

APPENDIX II

RESOURCES

MENOPAUSE

More than 1.5 million women go through the menopause every year, and millions more are experiencing symptoms of the climacteric as their ovarian function begins to decline. Support for the many changes taking place in your life during this transition is available to you through local menopause clinics and other organizations that offer both information and access to support groups. To find out if there are menopause workshops or groups in your area, contact your local YMCA, YWCA, American Red Cross, family or community service agencies, department of health or Planned Parenthood. If you want more information about menopause, or would like to join or start a support group for menopausal women, write or call this central clearing house:

> North American Menopause Society
> c/o Cleveland Menopause Clinic
> 29001 Cedar Road, No. 600
> Cleveland, OH 44124

WOMEN'S HEALTH CONCERNS

Every day, more and more attention—and research money—is being spent on the study of health care problems particular to women. There are several organizations and agencies prepared to share the information being gathered and advocate for continued research. Planned Parenthood provides literature, pamphlets, workshops, and film strips on a large variety of women's topics, including menopause. Contact your local branch to see what services are available in your area. The Women's Health Care Network is a national consumer organization devoted to women and health; members receive monthly newsletters on the latest developments in women's health care.

Planned Parenthood Federation of America
810 Seventh Avenue
New York, NY 10019
(212) 541-7800

The National Women's Health Network
1325 G Street NW
Washington, DC 20005
(202) 347-1140

GYNECOLOGICAL PROBLEMS

Menopause is just one of several gynecological conditions that affect women as they age; endometriosis is another. For more information about menopause, endometriosis, and other common—and not so common—gynecological conditions, contact:

Endometriosis Association Headquarters
8585 N 76th Place
Milwaukee, WI 53203
In the United States: (800) 992-ENDO
In Canada: (800) 426-2END

American College of Obstetricians
        and Gynecologists
Attention: Resource Center
409 12th Street SW
Washington, DC 20024-2188
(202) 638-5577

OSTEOPOROSIS

Brittle bones due to a lack of calcium and declining estrogen levels is a leading cause of disability and death in older American women, but, with proper care and attention, you can expect your bones to keep you upright and vigorous for as long as you live. For more information about osteoporosis and how you can prevent it from developing, write or call:

National Osteoporosis Foundation
1625 Eye Street NW, No. 822
Washington, DC 20006
(202) 223-2226

EXPANDING YOUR HORIZONS

Getting older means getting better more today than ever before. If you've reached the age of retirement or if you simply want to keep growing and learning, the following organizations can help you to find volunteer positions, educational opportunities, and employment.

> American Association of Retired Persons
> 1909 K Street NW
> Washington, DC 20049
> (202) 728-4450
>
> Association for Adult Education
> 1201 16th Street, Suite 230
> Washington, DC 20036
>
> Council of National Organizations for
>   Adult Education
> 174 Broadway, 17th Floor
> New York, NY 10019
>
> ACTION
> 806 Connecticut Avenue NW
> Washington, DC 20525

PLASTIC SURGERY

Every woman who thinks that plastic surgery may be an option for her has an obligation to learn as much about the procedure—and the surgeon—as possible. The following groups distribute free patient education brochures on various types of cosmetic surgery and provides a list of board-certified surgeons in your city.

> American Society of Plastic and
>   Reconstructive Surgeons
> 233 N Michigan Avenue, No. 1900
> Chicago, IL 60601
>
> American Academy of Facial and Plastic
>   Reconstructive Surgery
> 1110 Vermont Avenue NW
> Washington, DC 20005
> (202) 842-4500

SEXUALITY

Sexuality often becomes a major issue to a woman going through menopause. Although many aspects of sexual dysfunction related to menopause can be treated with estrogen and other medication, others require special attention from a professional trained in sex therapy. The following organization publishes a national register of Certified Sex Educators and Sex Therapists and will help you find a reputable sex therapist in your area.

American Association of Sex Educators,
Counselors, and Therapists
435 N Michigan Avenue, Suite 1717
Chicago, IL 60611
(312) 644-0828

SLEEP DISORDERS

Although most sleep problems associated with menopause can be easily treated with medication or self-help techniques, others are more intractable and need the attention of a sleep disorder professional. The Biofeedback Society can help you sort out the stresses and strains that may be preventing you from getting to sleep, while the American Sleep Disorders Association can direct you to the sleep disorder clinic nearest you for more specific help.

American Sleep Disorders Association
604 Second Street SW
Rochester, MN 55902
(507) 287-6006

Biofeedback Society of America
10200 West 44th Avenue
Wheatridge, CO 80033
(303) 422-8436

CANCER

The statistics remain alarming: breast cancer is the second leading cause of death in American women (the first is lung cancer), affecting one in every nine women. To learn more about how to prevent and how to treat breast and other cancers, write or call:

Breast Cancer Advisory Center
Box 224
Kensington, MD 20895
(301) 949-1132

Cancer Information Service, National Cancer Hotline
(800) 4-CANCER
In Hawaii: (800) 524-1234
In Alaska: (800) 638-6070
In Washington, DC: (202) 636-5700

DIABETES

One of the most common diseases among postmenopausal women—as well as older men—is type II diabetes. A killer often as silent and deadly as high blood pressure, diabetes causes or exacerbates heart and vessel disease and is the second leading cause of blindness (after accidents) in the United States. For more information about your risks for diabetes and how to prevent developing the disease or its side effects, write or call:

American Diabetes Association, Inc.
1660 Duke Street
Alexandria, VA 22314
(703) 549-1500

In Canada contact:
National Diabetes Association
78 Bond St.
Toronto, Canada M5B2JH
(416) 362-4440

CARDIOVASCULAR DISEASE

General information on prevention and treatment of cardiovascular disease is available from the following organizations; in addition, should you want to learn more about CPR and other emergency care procedures, the Red Cross offers classes in many communities. Please note that there are branches of the Red Cross in every major city in the country. The American Heart Association, with branches in every major city across the country, is a font of information about all aspects of cardiovascular disease. Diet and exercise plans to lower blood pressure and other cardiovascular ailments, research papers describing the latest medical breakthroughs in diagnosis and treatment, and pamphlets on symptoms of heart disease and stroke are also available through this organization.

> American Red Cross
> 17th and D Streets NW
> Washington, DC 20006
> (301) 737-8300

> The American Heart Association
> 7320 Greenville Avenue
> Dallas, TX 75231
> (214) 750-5551

In Canada, please write:
> Heart and Stroke Foundation of Canada
> 160 George Street, Suite 200
> Ottawa, Ontario K1N9M2

PHYSICAL FITNESS

Physical fitness is more than a fad, it's a sure-fire way to lessen the risk of osteoporosis, hypertension and other cardiovascular diseases, and reduce stress and tension. In almost every town in the country, health clubs and spas, not to mention the old reliable YWCA, can get you in shape in just a few months of hard work. For more information, please write:

> The President's Council on Physical Fitness and Sports
> 400 Sixth Street NW
> Washington, DC 20201

> American Alliance for Health, Physical Education
>   and Recreation
> 1201 16th Street NW
> Washington, DC 20036

STOP SMOKING NOW!

Many people need encouragement and help to stop smoking. The organizations listed below can give you advice on how to stop smoking on your own or recommend reputable medical or psychological techniques:

> American Cancer Society/National Office
> 19 West 56th Street
> New York City 10001
> (212) 586-8700

Office of Cancer Communications
National Cancer Institute
Bethesda, MD 20205
(301) 496-4000

American Lung Association
1740 Broadway
New York City 10019
(212) 315-8700

In Canada contact:
Canadian Cancer Society
77 Bloor Street, Suite 1701
Toronto, Ontario M5S3A1
(416) 961-7223

CONCERNS OF THE AGING

Although menopause affects women as young as thirty-five
or forty, most women experience this transition in their fifties
and are only just beginning to think about their future after
retirement. At the same time, they may have questions about
how to care for their own aging parents once they can no longer
take care of themselves. If you have questions about Medicare,
home nursing care, or any other issue associated with aging and
illness, many national and state agencies can help you. Check
your telephone directory for local agencies or contact:

Medicaid/Medicare
Health Financing Administration
Department of Health and Human Services
Washington, DC 20201
(202) 245-0312

National Council of Senior Citizens
925 15th Street NW
Washington, DC 20005
(202) 347-8800

American Association for Retired Persons
1909 K Street NW
Washington, DC 20049
(202) 872-4700

Gray Panthers
3700 Chestnut Street
Philadelphia, PA 19104

GLOSSARY

Absorptiometry: a medical test to measure the density of bone that uses low-energy radioisotopes.

Adrenal glands: small, pyramid-shaped glands situated on top of each kidney largely responsible for controlling sugar and salt metabolism. They also secrete the androgen hormones and small amounts of estrogen and progestogen.

Adrenaline: neurotransmitter produced by the adrenal gland that is released in response to fear, heightened emotion, or physiological stress.

Amenorrhea: lack of menstruation.

Amino acids: the nitrogen-containing building blocks of protein used by the body to form muscle and other tissue.

Androgenic: a substance or hormone that produces male or masculine characteristics.

Androgens: hormones secreted in small amounts by the adrenal glands that produce male or masculine characteristics.

Androstenedione: an androgen secreted by the adrenal glands that is converted by fat cells into a form of estrogen.

Androsterone: an androgen.

Angiotensin: a substance in the blood that causes blood vessels to narrow or constrict, thereby raising blood pressure. The level of angiotensin rises following ovulation, which exacerbates fluid accumulation and bloating.

Atherosclerosis: "hardening of the arteries;" a disease in which fatty plaque develops on the anterior walls of the arteries, eventually obstructing blood flow.

Atrophic vaginitis: inflammation of the vaginal tissue caused by thinning of the vaginal wall due to a lack of estrogen.

Bellergal: medication used to treat hot flashes in women who are not candidates for estrogen therapy.

Biopsy: removal and microscopic examination of a small sample of tissue from the body to make a diagnosis.

Calcium: mineral essential to building and maintaining bones and teeth, and instrumental in blood clotting and the proper function of muscles, nerves, and heart.

Cancer: abnormal growth of cells that may destroy the body's vital organs; there are more than one hundred different types of cancer.

Cervical canal polyps: benign growths in the endocervical canal that may protrude through the cervix and cause abnormal bleeding.

Cervix: the neck, or narrow part, of the uterus that protrudes into the vaginal cavity.

Cholesterol: a fatty substance needed by the body to form cell membranes; made in the liver and essential to production of sex hormones, nerve function, and other processes; excessive consumption of dietary cholesterol (found in animal products) raises blood cholesterol levels, which may lead to atherosclerosis.

Climacteric: the ten years or so before a woman experiences her last menstrual period during which time her monthly hormonal cycle begins to change from a reproductive to nonreproductive state.

Clonidine: a medication usually used to treat high blood pressure and known to provide some relief for hot flashes in women unable to take estrogen.

Collagen: a fibrous protein that forms a connective tissue supporting the skin, bone, tendons, and cartilage; injections of collagen are sometimes used to fill in wrinkles, burns, and scars.

Colposcopy: a medical procedure in which a telescope-like instrument is used to look at the cervix and vagina to locate abnormal cells.

Conception: the fertilization of an egg by sperm, resulting in pregnancy.

Conjugated estrogen: a mixture of estrogens, either natural or artificial, that can be prescribed to relieve symptoms of menopause and to treat failure to ovulate.

Contraceptive: an agent or device used to prevent conception.

Corpus luteum: the small yellow organ that forms in the ovary following ovulation from the ruptured ovarian follicle; produces the hormone progesterone responsible for counteracting the build-up of estrogen in the uterine lining during the second half of the menstrual cycle.

Corticosteriods: hormones produced by the outer layer of the adrenal gland that are instrumental in the proper metabolism of carbohydrates and proteins, the function of the heart, lungs, muscles, kidneys, and other organs.

Cortisol: the principal corticosteroid responsible for helping to regulate blood sugar, blood pressure, and bone growth. Also known as hydrocortisone.

Cortisone: a hormone isolated from the adrenal gland or produced synthetically that is converted to cortisol in the body.

Cyst: a closed sac that contains a liquid or semi-solid substance; many women develop harmless cysts in the breast or ovary; other cysts may be a sign of an abnormal infection or tumor.

Dilation and curettage (D & C): a surgical procedure in which the cervix is dilated and the lining of the uterus is scraped; used to treat and diagnose diseases of the uterus, to remove polyps and other small growths, and to correct heavy vaginal bleeding; may also be used as an abortion technique or to remove remaining pregnancy tissue after a miscarriage.

Dysfunctional uterine bleeding: uterine or vaginal bleeding that takes place in the absence of ovulation; usually attributed to abnormal or irregular production of hormones by the ovary.

Dysmenorrhea: painful menstrual periods common to about ten percent of women.

Endocrine system: ductless glands and other structures that secrete hormones into the bloodstream; the pituitary, thyroid, adrenal, and hypothalamus glands, the ovaries, kidneys, small intestine, lungs, and heart also produce hormones.

Endometriosis: common disorder in which some endometrial cells that normally line the uterus escape into the pelvic cavity and form clusters on other organs, such as the ovaries, fallopian tubes, and colon. These cells may respond to hormonal stimulus during each menstrual cycle and become engorged with blood, causing severe pain.

Endometrium: the lining of the internal surface of the uterus in which the fertilized ovum is implanted but which is shed during menstruation if conception has not occurred.

Estradiol: a form of natural human estrogen secreted mostly by the ovarian follicle; responsible for the development of secondary sex characteristics in teenage girls and promoting the growth of the endometrium during the first part of the menstrual cycle.

Estrogen: a group of female hormones responsible for the development of secondary sex traits, such as the breasts and menstruation; produced in the ovaries, adrenal glands, and both the fetus and placenta.

Estrogen replacement therapy (ERT): the use of estrogen alone to treat menopause (as opposed to hormone replacement therapy).

Fallopian tubes: long slender tubes, extending from each side of the uterus and ending near the ovaries, that pick up the egg after ovulation; fertilization normally occurs within these tubes.

Fibrocystic breast disease: a common benign breast condition in which an abundance of cysts arises from the glands within the breast tissue.

Fibroid tumor: mostly benign uterine tumors made up of smooth muscle cells; common after the age of 35; large, fast-growing fibroids may require surgery.

Fibrosarcoma: a cancerous fibroid tumor.

Follicles: the egg-forming cells in the ovaries.

Follicular stimulating hormone (FSH): a hormone secreted by the pituitary gland prompting the maturation of an egg within the ovary; controlled by estrogen produced by the egg; rises to very high levels when the ovaries no longer produce estrogen. An elevated FSH is an indication of menopause.

Formication: relatively rare menopausal symptom in which a woman feels a tingling sensation, as if insects are crawling on her skin.

Gallbladder: a sac located on the underside of the liver that stores the bile helpful in the digestion of fats.

Gland: any organ that produces and secretes a chemical substance used by another part of the body.

Gonads: primary sex glands: ovaries in the female, testes in the male.

Gonadotropin releasing hormone (GnRH): a hormone produced by the hypothalamus that stimulates the pituitary gland to produce follicle stimulating hormone and luteinizing hormone.

HDL-cholesterol: high-density lipoprotein cholesterol that carries cholesterol away from the tissue for excretion from the body; also known as the "good cholesterol."

Hormones: chemicals produced by the endocrine glands or tissue that affect other organs; influence growth, sexual development, metabolism, behavior, and other essential human activities; also known as "chemical messengers."

Hormone replacement therapy (HRT): the use of both estrogen and progesterone, and possibly an androgen, to replace the hormones no longer produced after menopause.

Hot flash: a common menopausal symptom consisting of a feeling of intense heat coupled with redness and perspiration.

Hypothalamus: the part of the brain that works with the pituitary to control the reproductive system and other human functions.

Hysterectomy: surgical removal of the uterus.

Kegel exercises: exercises used to strengthen the muscles around the urethra, bladder, and rectum to increase muscle tone.

Laparoscopy: a surgical procedure in which a fiberoptic endoscope is inserted into the umbilicus to look directly at the uterus, fallopian tubes, and ovaries.

LDL-cholesterol: low-density lipoprotein cholesterol that deposits cholesterol in the blood vessels; the "bad cholesterol."

Lipids: fatty substances consisting of cholesterol and triglycerides.

Luteinization: the development of the corpus luteum within a ruptured follicle following ovulation.

Luteinizing hormone (LH): hormone produced by the pituitary gland that works together with the follicle stimulating hormone (FSH) to stimulate the ovary to secrete estrogen. High levels of estrogen cause a surge of LH, which stimulates ovulation.

Mammogram: an x-ray of the breasts to screen for breast cancer.

Menarche: a woman's first menstruation period.

Menopause: the end of a woman's ability to reproduce; a woman's last menstrual period.

Menstrual cycle: a woman's monthly cycle, characterized by hormonal changes that thicken the endometrium to prepare the body for pregnancy; if pregnancy does not occur, the endometrium is shed during menstruation and a new cycle begins; average length of cycle is twenty-eight days.

Menses: the monthly period of uterine bleeding and shedding of endometrium; also called menstruation or menstrual period; lasts about four or five days.

Myomectomy: surgical procedure to remove fibroid tumors, particularly from the uterus.

Oligomenorrhea: infrequent menstrual bleeding due to irregular ovulation.

Oligoovulation: irregular ovulation.

Oophorectomy: surgical removal of the ovaries; unilateral oophorectomy is removal of one ovary, bilateral oophorectomy is removal of both ovaries.

Oral contraceptive: oral steroid drug for birth control; usually consists of a combination of progestogen and estrogen.

Osteoporosis: the condition in which bones become thin and porous as a result of calcium loss.

Ovarian cyst: a saclike structure in the ovary that causes an enlargement of the ovary.

Ovarian failure: the inability of the ovary to produce estrogen; also known as menopause.

Ovary: the female reproductive glands that produce eggs and the sex hormones estrogen and progesterone.

Ovulation: the periodic rupture of a mature follicle and dispatch of the egg from the ovary.

Pap smear (Papanicolaou test): a medical examination of cells from the cervix or bronchi to diagnose cancerous and precancerous conditions.

Pelvic inflammatory disease (PID): serious infection of the reproductive organs.

Perimenopause: the years prior to the last menstrual period.

Pituitary gland: pea-sized gland located between and behind the eyes in the base of the brain; secretes hormones to control many other important glands in the body, including ovaries, thyroid, and adrenal glands; controlled by the hypothalamus.

Polyp: growth arising from the mucus membrane of a body cavity; common in the uterine cavity; may cause abnormal bleeding.

Premature menopause: ovarian failure that occurs before the age of thirty-five to forty.

Premenstrual syndrome (PMS): physical and emotional symptoms associated with the menstrual cycle.

Progesterone: hormone produced by the corpus luteum after a woman ovulates; prepares the endometrium for pregnancy; fall in progesterone production initiates the menstrual period.

Progestin, progestogen: hormones related to the hormone progesterone released by the corpus luteum, placenta, or adrenal cortex; have progesterone-like effects; used in conjunction with estrogen in hormone replacement therapy.

Puberty: developmental stage during which secondary sex characteristics manifest themselves and reproductive organs become functional; usually accompanied by rapid physical growth.

Senile urethral syndrome: symptoms of urinary frequency, urgency, and pain on urination due to the thinning of the urethra from lack of estrogen.

Steroid hormones: the sex hormones and hormones of the adrenal cortex including corticosteriods, mineralcorticoids, androgen, estrogen, and progesterone.

Stress incontinence: loss of urine associated with an increase in intra-abdominal pressure, such as in coughing or sneezing.

Tamoxifen: drug that counters effects of estrogen; used to treat advanced breast cancer in premenopausal women whose tumors are estrogen-dependent; also used to reduce discomfort caused by fibrocystic breast disease.

Testes: male sex glands enclosed in scrotum that produce the male sex hormone testosterone, as well as sperm.

Testosterone: male hormone produced by the testes in men; women's ovaries also produce a small amount of testosterone.

Thyroid gland: large, butterfly-shaped gland located in front of and on each side of the trachea that secretes thyroxin and other hormones responsible for numerous metabolic processes; essential for the regulation of the body's metabolism, including heart beat, temperature control, and other essential processes.

Unopposed estrogen therapy: treatment for menopausal symptoms that consists of estrogen alone, without progesterone.

Urethra: membranous canal that carries urine from the bladder to the exterior of the body; sensitive to estrogen in women.

Urethritis: inflammation or infection of the urethra.

Uterine prolapse: condition in which the uterus descends into the lower part of the vagina or outside the vaginal opening.

Uterus: hollow muscular female organ in which the fetus develops; consists of the body, the cervix, and the endometrium; also known as the womb.

Vagina: the canal in the female extending from the vulva to the cervix; extremely sensitive to lack of estrogen at menopause.

Vaginitis: inflammation or infection of vagina often caused by lack of estrogen.

Vasomotor instability: rapid rise in body temperature accompanied by perspiration caused by fluctuating hormone levels; also known as hot flashes.

Vulva: woman's external genital organs including the mons pubis, labia majora, labia minora, clitoris, and other structures.

INDEX

Abdominal cramps, 77
Abdominal hysterectomies, 104, 145
Absorptiometry, 58
Adrenal glands, 18
Aerobic exercise, 161–63, 164
Age spots, 131
Aging, 26, 55, 64, 189
AIDS, 126
Alcohol consumption, 56, 122, 154–55
Amen, 74
Amenorrhea, 94
Anaerobic exercise, 161–62
Androgens, 18, 22, 41
Anemia, 102
Angiotensinogen, 71
Antacids, 152
Antibiotics, 139
Anticoagulants, 57
Antidepressants, 116
Antifungal drugs, 139
Antigravitational exercises, 166–67
Antihormonal therapy, 99
Anti-oxidants, 149
Arthritis, 109–10
Aspirin, 110
Atelectasis, 54
Atherosclerosis, 11, 60, 61–62, 85
Autoimmune disorders, 24

Baths, 130
Behavior therapy, 123
Bellegral (phenobarbital), 77
Beta-endorphin release, 87, 116
Bilateral oophorectomy, 24, 28, 97, 105–6
Biofeedback, 123
Birth control, 36, 68, 82, 126
Birth defects, 67–68
Bleeding, excessive uterine, 103
Blood clotting, 62, 82–83
Blood lipids, test for, 171–72
Blood pressure test, 172–73
Blood tests, 32, 79, 171–72, 174–75
Body hair, 18, 118–19
Bone-building exercises, 166–67
Bone density, 56, 79, 165–66, 175
Bone fractures, 49
Bone regeneration, 50
Bone-sparing drugs, 59–60

Breast augmentation/reduction, 112
Breast cancer, 68, 81–82
Breast changes, self-help strategies for, 111–12
Breast examinations, 79, 176–77
Breastfeeding, 50, 150
Breast swelling/tenderness, 77
Buccal estrogen, 73

Caffeine, 56, 116, 122
Calcitonin, 51–52, 59
Calcium, 50–52, 57, 58, 148, 150–52
Calisthenics, 166
Calories, 143, 155–59
Cancer, 36
  breast, 68, 81–82
  endometrial, 67, 70, 74, 80–81, 101
  estrogen-dependent, 82, 98–99
  ovarian, 98
  resources for, 186–87
Carbohydrates, 143–44, 157
Carcinogens, 80
Cardiovascular disease, 25, 26, 60–66, 85, 90, 149, 153–54, 163–65, 187–88
Catapres, 76
Chemical oophorectomy, 100
Chemical peels, 132
Chemotherapy, 25, 94–95
Cholesterol, 61–63, 79, 145–47, 171–72
Chorionic gonadotrophin, 20
Chromosomes, 17, 25
Circulatory system, 61–62
Climacteric, 15–16, 21–22
Clonidine, 76
Clothing, and hot flashes, 121
Collagen, 39, 40, 49, 52, 132
Conjugated estrogens, 71, 82–83
Constipation, 54
Corpus luteum, 20
Cortical bone, 49
Cortisol, 122
Cortisone preparations, 57
Cosmetic surgery, 132–33
Crown replacement, 113
Curretabs, 74
Cycle regimen for hormone replacement therapy, 75–76
Cystocele, 137

Dairy products, 144–45
D&C (dilation and curettage), 102, 103–4, 178
Densitometry, 58
Dental care, 54, 112–14
Depilatories, 118
Depression, 27–28, 39, 77, 114–17
Dermabrasion, 132
Dermatological changes, 26, 39–41, 86
DES (diethylstilbestrol), 67–68
Diabetes, 17, 65, 187
Diastole stage, 173
Didronel, 59
Diet, 140
  alcohol intake, 56, 122, 154–55
  calcium in, 150–52
  and cardiovascular disease, 111
  cholesterol in, 146–47
  dairy products in, 144–45
  essential nutrients for balanced diet, 142–44
  fad diets, 157
  fat in, 145–46
  to fight sadness, 116
  iron in, 153–54
  for menopausal women, 23–24, 141–42
  sodium in, 152–53
  vitamins and minerals, 147–54
  and weight loss, 155–59
Diethylstilbestrol (DES), 67–68
Diuretics, 57
Douches, 138–39
Dowager's hump, 48, 53
Dysuria, 43

Educational opportunities, 185
Elavil, 116
Electrocardiogram, 79
Electroconvulsive therapy, 116
Electrolysis, 119
Emboli, 82–83
Emotional changes, 27–28, 45–47, 87
Employment, resources for, 185
Endocrine system, 17
Endometrial biopsy, 79, 178–79

ABOUT THE AUTHORS

LOIS JOVANOVIC, M.D., is a clinical associate professor at USC. She is board certified in both internal medicine and endocrinology. On the editorial board of eight medical journals, Dr. Jovanovic is the co-author of *Hormones: the Woman's Answerbook* with Genell J. Subak-Sharpe.

SUZANNE LEVERT is a writer and editor who specializes in health-related subjects. Her recent titles include *Parkinson's Disease: A Complete Guide for Patients and Care Givers* and *If It Runs in the Family: Hypertension and Diabetes*.